Understanding
Obesity

Understanding Obesity

Dr. Lance Levy

FIREFLY BOOKS

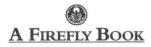

A FIREFLY BOOK

Published by Firefly Books Ltd. 2000

First Printing

U.S. Cataloging-in-Publication Data

Levy, Lance.
    Understanding obesity / Lance Levy.—1st ed.

[192]p. : ill. : cm.—(Your Personal Health)
Summary: Causes and treatments of obesity.
ISBN 1-55209-479-0 (pbk.)

1 Obesity. 2. Obesity—Psychological aspects. I. Title. II. Series

616.398   21   2000   CIP

Published in the United States in 2000 by
Firefly Books (U.S.) Inc.
P.O. Box 1338, Ellicott Station
Buffalo, New York, USA
14205

Published in Canada in 2000 by Key Porter Books Limited.

Electronic formatting: Heidy Lawrance Associates
Design: Peter Maher

The publisher has made every effort to contact the copyright holders of extracts reproduced in this book. We would be pleased to have any additional information regarding this material.

Printed and bound in Canada

*The best thing I ever did
in my life was to be
father to my two amazing sons,
Harrison and Jack Levy.*

This book is dedicated to them.

Contents

Introduction: There's No "One-Size-Fits-All" Method for Losing Weight

This book is intended as a guide for anyone who is overweight and looking for sensible approaches for dealing with the problem. In these pages I describe what we currently know about the causes and management of obesity. We are on the verge of having a useful understanding of the complex reasons why people become obese, and I discuss these in some depth. It is only fair to warn you, however, that completely successful methods of weight loss are still far off, and successful long-term treatments are difficult to devise.

Let us start with two basic questions. First, what is obesity? And second, why should anyone worry about it? The World Health Organization's criteria for Body Mass Index (BMI) have recently been adopted as the universal standard for defining levels of overweight and obesity. (The Body Mass Index is your weight in kilograms divided by the square of your height expressed in centimeters.) A Body Mass Index of less than 18.5 signifies malnutrition or significant underweight, a BMI from 18.5 to 24 is normal, from 25 to 29 is overweight, and above 30 indicates obesity. Though using BMI alone as a measure of weight problems has its limitations (as will be discussed later), according to the recent Canadian Heart Health Survey, approximately 44 percent of men and 25 percent of women have a BMI of 25 to 29 (overweight). Thirteen percent of men and 14 percent of women have a BMI over 30 (obese). Therefore, if we take a BMI of 24.9 as the cutoff above which an individual is too heavy, 57 percent of men are overweight or obese and 39 percent of women are in the same category. Thus, fully 48 percent of our adult population are excessively heavy. In the United States, using slightly different cut-offs for BMI, 31 percent of adults have a BMI of 25 to 30, and 21 percent have a BMI above 30 and so are obese.

There is also a very disturbing trend in the development of weight problems in our children. In 1981, 15 percent of children were overweight or obese, while in 1998, 24 percent were overweight or obese. (The concept of an "ideal" weight raises further questions, but for now let's accept that there is an approximate "healthy" weight for most people.)

The reason we need to be concerned is that excess weight is the cause of more illness than virtually any other medical condition. Even in the poorest countries, obesity is becoming epidemic, causing significant ill health from diabetes and heart disease where these were relatively rare thirty years ago. In the western industrialized countries, many more people will have to see a doctor because of complications arising from overweight than will develop cancer! For example, 80 percent of adult-onset diabetes occurs in people who are overweight or obese. Diabetes, heart and vascular disease, high-blood pressure (hypertension), gallbladder disease, arthritis, sleep apnea (a condition where people fail to breathe adequately during sleep), and gastrointestinal ailments are just some of the health problems that can afflict the overweight person.

Not surprisingly, the medical and socio-economic costs of obesity are high. Of all the health-care dollars spent in the United States in 1990, 6.8 percent (about $34 billion) were spent on the physical and psychological treatments directly associated with obesity. In Canada, 2.4 percent of the health care budget was spent for these problems. It is important to note that these costs are for the treatment of obesity-related problems (such as heart disease) only and do not include the additional costs that occur where, for example, wages are lost due to obesity-linked illness such as arthritis, high blood pressure, and early death. From a public-health perspective, allowing this illness to remain so poorly researched and treated has been a very costly mistake for governments. The fact that governments have begun to approve weight-control drugs for the long-term management of serious obesity is a step in the right direction. Another positive step is the search for weight-management approaches that will work with children and adolescents who will undoubtedly become fat adults if left untreated.

Obesity has increased in the past decade. There are a number of possible reasons why this is so. Several that I am particularly interested in are the use of poorly devised diets, the effects of advertising on dietary food choices, food manipulation to enhance palatability, and the role of stress in promoting weight gain. As an example of the first, the increase in overweight may be in part linked to the dietary approaches in most common use, such as the advocacy of quite low-fat diets and diets that are more than 500 to 750 calories below that needed for weight maintenance (for example, a 1200-calorie diet for a man weighing 300 pounds (136 kg) whose calorie requirement for maintaining weight would be roughly 3500 calories). This may seem contradictory, but as I explain later, low-fat diets (those with fewer than 25 percent of their calories from fat) and excessively deprivational diets can encourage weight to be regained.

It is true, too, that our society is becoming increasingly "hostile" to sensible food management, because the food industry has invested heavily to make foods as flavorful and appealing as possible and to encourage us, through advertising, to eat when we are not hungry. When food is very tasty we eat more. Since it may also be high in fat and we are not burning enough calories, we gain weight. Also, we are under more stress now than twenty years ago, and people often eat in an attempt to relieve stress and maintain energy. Last but not least, as a society we are less active now than in previous decades. Our children are particularly inactive compared to their counterparts of forty years ago. Inactivity makes it much harder to balance food intake against calories expended.

I have looked after patients with weight-control problems for the past fourteen years. The weight-loss efforts of most of these people were complicated by unrecognized and usually untreated or partially treated medical problems such as those mentioned above. Managing weight loss with a patient is one of the most challenging projects a doctor and patient can work on together. There are more failures than successes because obesity is such a complex problem. Because no two overweight people are overweight for the same reasons, simple dietary instruction and advice such as "be more active" are rarely effective. In-depth assessment and treatment are needed, particularly when a person has been overweight for a long time or is very overweight.

It is all too easy to spend a lot of time and money trying to lose weight in ways that will not work or that are almost certainly harmful, either because they predispose the dieter to more weight gain later or simply because they are unsafe. North Americans spent tens of billions of dollars last year on various weight-loss approaches, but many of the people who go to a commercial diet center regain the weight they lost within two years and often end up heavier than they were before they dieted. Research shows that only about thirty-five out of every hundred moderately obese people who undertake one of the best medically devised weight-loss plans will lose 15 percent of their starting body weight and maintain that loss after two years. Claims that are better than this are unlikely to be reliable.

The approach described in this book is radically different from that of most weight-loss programs. Instead of offering a "one-size-fits-all" recipe for losing weight, it looks at weight loss as a highly individual matter. Weight management is a complex task involving both emotional and physical factors. This book outlines some of the reasons why weight loss is hard and the physics behind why we gain or lose weight. It explains the various methods of medically evaluating a patient and of managing the weight-loss process. All weight-loss strategies have to be individualized if they are to work. Medically supervised drug management of appetite is an important part of treating serious obesity, and a chapter is dedicated to this topic.

Problems with mood, such as anxiety, depression, and chronic unhappiness states (dysthymia), are very common. Patients often believe that their mood will improve as weight loss proceeds, but though a person may temporarily feel less depressed or unhappy while he or she is losing weight, long-term improvement in mood is rarely the result of weight loss alone. One chapter explains why weight-loss approaches that ignore mood problems will generally not succeed, while approaches that treat mood problems and weight problems together can be helpful. In my experience, the majority of overweight people succeed in losing weight only when they are feeling more positive about life.

In keeping with the focus on the *person* rather than the *diet*, this book reviews several well-known diets but cannot honestly advocate any one of them. The reasons why we don't promote diets—even a *Canada's Food Guide* 1500-calorie diet—are simple.

Our studies on dietary awareness show that obese patients can usually identify helpful changes they could make in their diets. Almost any of these changes, if put into practice over the long term, would result in sustained and adequate weight loss. Therefore the real challenge in helping a person lose weight is in understanding *why* that intelligent person cannot make these changes. Understanding why people are not making changes is more important than counting their calorie intake. It is not very helpful to coach adults on how many teaspoons of mayonnaise they should use in their tuna sandwich. In fact, doing so merely proves to them that you don't really understand why they have weight problems. It is more constructive to help people identify the things that are preventing them from eating properly than to lecture them on diet theory. Everyone knows that to achieve weight loss over time a person needs to consume fewer calories than are burned. It sounds as though losing weight should be a simple, almost mechanical process. In fact, however, people cannot reduce their calorie intake over the long term until they understand how to control their appetite. The choices we make about what food to eat, the timing of meals, the balance of protein, fat, and carbohydrate, and activity level all affect appetite. Above all, patients need to learn how to interpret and respond to appetite signals and to find ways to increase activity level. The diet theory can wait till later.

Every strategy for weight loss is based on a particular philosophy. If there were one that was completely right, I wouldn't be writing this book. I believe that any weight-loss book can be helpful if it does two things well. First, its suggestions must be rooted in the actual experiences of people who have struggled with overweight and tried different approaches. Second, it must approach weight-control issues as true medical problems, not just a matter of summoning up a little self-restraint and willpower.

My weight-loss strategy is based on my observation that you will not succeed in losing weight and keeping it off until your medical/psychological problems are treated and improvement has been secured, and your thinking about weight loss has changed in the following ways:

1. First, you must find a meaningful, personal, "core" reason to lose weight. Here is an example.

   One of my patients, "Kathy" (not her real name), a nurse in her thirties, weighed over 320 pounds (136 kg). Over a three-year period we tried every weight-loss approach I knew, including various medications. She had been managed very well for a bipolar disorder (abrupt, extreme mood swings), and had been put on supplemental air for sleep apnea (a condition where a person does not breathe enough during sleep). Nevertheless, despite all her efforts, she did not lose weight. She had such bad arthritis in both knees that she was likely to be in a wheelchair within five years. As a last resort, I suggested stomach surgery and referred her to a surgeon. (I add that I recommend gastric surgery for obesity only when I am persuaded that no medical option remains, and that the patient will suffer serious medical consequences from the obesity. I must also be satisfied that the patient is psychologically fit for this procedure.) Just after I made the referral, the patient began to lose weight, and in five months lost nearly 50 pounds (22 kg). What, I asked her, had suddenly changed in her thinking? She said that with the referral to a surgeon, she realized on a very intense, deep level, that her freedom, her career, and indeed her whole life were about to go up in smoke because of her obesity. She said that she was totally determined *never* to end up in that wheelchair. Finally, she had a reason to lose weight that really meant something to her. The things she valued most deeply were being put at risk by her obesity, and she had come far along enough in her psychotherapy to finally confront that reality honestly.

2. Second, you must accept that there is a cost to everything, including health.

When other aspects of their lives are difficult, people may feel that the effort needed to maintain good health is too much for them. But when they come to appreciate that staying healthy is a prerequisite for holding onto the things they have worked hard to achieve, they can succeed in losing weight and keeping it off. Although we cannot subordinate all other aspects of life to health issues, we do have to decide to adjust our priorities to protect health. For example, building time for physical activity into the day is essential even if it means saying no to other responsibilities—including even some work-related ones.

3. Third, you must feel capable of dealing with the fears, insecurities, or negative thoughts that prevent you from changing.

Think of the word "fear" as an acronym that stands for *Fantasy Experienced As Reality*. Many of the obstacles my patients report that prevent them from changing their lifestyles are more imaginary than real. The "obstacle" is that they see a required change as dangerous. For example, they may be reluctant to ask for flexible hours at work in order to take an hour's walk at lunch break, imagining that the boss will think them too demanding and refuse, or become angry and punitive. They may remember similar events when they were children or adolescents and couldn't adequately explain their needs, forgetting that as adults they are very capable of making their case.

Becoming less afraid allows them to reorganize their day without feeling guilty about it. When they do this, most people find that friends and colleagues support their efforts. The resistance they worried about does not materialize.

As I said early in this introduction, the treatment of weight problems is a complex matter. This is partly because each person is unique and partly because there are so many physiological and psychological dimensions to our use of food. In the rest of this book, I look at different aspects of the problem in more detail. The next two chapters describe the eating patterns that most commonly accompany weight problems and examine some of the reasons why people can become locked into such patterns. Three chapters are then given over to aspects of the physiology of weight gain, and another chapter to the need to treat medical conditions that can make it hard for people to lose weight. In two subsequent chapters, I evaluate some approaches to weight loss that are currently in use and then discuss my own approach, which focuses on finding out what works best for the individual. The last four chapters deal with a variety of topics, including the use of drugs in weight management, childhood obesity, controlling weight gain under a variety of special conditions (such as pregnancy), and more invasive forms of treatment (such as gastric surgery).

It is my hope that the information that follows will provide helpful insights into the physical and emotional aspects of weight loss and weight gain, and will enable you, the reader, to find answers and solutions to fit your own individual circumstances.

1. It's How (and Why) You Eat, as Well as What You Eat: "Disordered Eating" and Weight Gain

One of the first points to consider when trying to manage a weight problem is not *what* you eat but your daily eating pattern. In my experience, many overweight people are locked into a pattern of "disordered eating." I hasten to add that disordered eating is not the same thing as an eating disorder. The term "eating disorder" has come to be used incorrectly to describe the behavior of a person who is routinely overeating or who feels he or she is a food addict. However, such people suffer from "disordered eating" rather than the psychiatric conditions known as "eating disorders" (Appendix 1). In fact, eating disorders have specific diagnostic criteria and are quite different from excessive or even compulsive eating. A few specific definitions will be helpful here.

The two eating disorders most commonly diagnosed are anorexia nervosa and bulimia nervosa.

Anorexia Nervosa

Anorexia nervosa is a condition in which people restrict their food intake so much that they suffer a marked loss of weight. Furthermore, they refuse to maintain a normal body weight and are intensely afraid of gaining weight or of being fat. Their need to restrict food and their preoccupation with being fat continues even while they lose more weight and become emaciated. These people have a disturbance in the way they experience their body shape, typically seeing themselves as grossly fat when they are actually skinny. In females who are past puberty, menstrual periods cease. There are several subtypes of anorexia nervosa, characterized by the different methods sufferers use to keep weight very low.

The most common problem for such patients is the effect of malnutrition on their ability to function mentally and physically at home and at work. There is progressive erosion of their ability to do physical work, and their ability to think clearly and concentrate also deteriorates. As well, a common symptom of the illness is strong denial that anything is wrong. My experience is that patients with anorexia usually know at some level that they are in trouble, but fear of gaining weight prevents them from admitting there is a problem. They tend to seek treatment only when their family and friends force them to. Anorexia is thought of as a disease of young women, and 90 percent of those affected as teenagers are female. However, 25 percent of patients who are forty-five or older are men. Anorexia is a serious illness at any time of life, but is especially lethal in the elderly.

Bulimia Nervosa

Bulimia nervosa is diagnosed when a person has experienced recurrent episodes of binge eating and uses extreme measures to get rid of the excess calories. Binge eating has very specific characteristics and is different from simple overeating. Binge eaters are usually aware of craving a certain food or foods. Once they begin to eat they feel powerless to stop until one of the following things happens: they become painfully full, run out of food, fall asleep, are interrupted by someone, or vomit. Binge eaters also try to avoid weight gain by getting rid of food binged through such measures as inducing vomiting, using laxatives, fasting, and hyper-exercising.

Both anorexic and bulimic patients may experience serious mood changes over time. Depression is common but may develop gradually. It is often not noticed because patients are so preoccupied with their weight problem. It has been observed that depression is a common cause of the eating disorder and that starving or binge eating are designed to minimize the pain of the mood state.

If you believe you are experiencing these symptoms, see your doctor for a full assessment. Like obesity, an eating disorder is a true medical problem, not a character flaw! The sooner it is diagnosed the sooner the person can be helped.

Compulsive Overeating: Binge Eating Disorder

A third disorder that is much more common than is generally realized has recently been classified as "binge eating disorder." Here, sufferers feel the compulsion to eat and can't stop until they are either painfully full, run out of food, are interrupted, or fall asleep. The mood problems seen in bulimia and anorexia are also present, but because such symptoms as vomiting or abuse of laxatives are absent, many people with this problem feel they don't have an eating disorder. To relieve attacks of compulsive binge eating, medications such as Prozac are often prescribed.

Disordered Eating

Disordered eating, which is much more common than the eating disorders just described, is not a psychiatric disorder. We all overeat from time to time and will feel uncomfortably full after such an episode. When we routinely have trouble scheduling meals, eat more fast food or junk food than we know is good for us, or miss meals, eating has become disorganized and weight control will suffer. Disordered eating happens when various medical problems, life events, or emotional states interfere with our awareness of, or ability to respond appropriately to, signals for hunger and fullness. Unlike the eating disordered, a person with disorganized eating does not have a feeling of being out of control with food.

"Kathy," the nurse I described in the introduction, suffered from disordered eating. She was so busy trying to please her friends and co-workers that she pushed all her own needs aside. When she felt overtired and pressured by work, and also when she was anxious, she would feel "hungry" and would overeat without understanding the underlying cause of her hunger—a need to regain energy and reduce stress. In her case, she had difficulty realizing when she was genuinely hungry and when she had actually had enough food. The result: difficulty in regulating her food intake, leading to obesity.

The following case histories illustrate disordered eating further.

Case 1: Eating to Minimize Distress and Maintain Energy Level. Unrecognized Depression

"Kelly" (again, not her real name) is a high school teacher in her mid-thirties who came to see me for help with obesity. She was 5 feet, 5 inches (165 cm) tall and weighed 312 pounds (141 kg).

She had a history of being unable to keep weight off ever since her mid-teens. At various times in the past she had been able to lose up to 60 pounds (27 kg) by following a commercial diet plan, but had always gained the weight back, and more. Once, in her early twenties, she had gone so far as to have surgery to have her stomach stapled in an effort to control her weight. She had lost about 30 percent of her starting weight, but regained all of it and more over the years. (I will discuss stomach surgery and obesity in more detail later. For now, I will just say that with complicating factors such as emotional issues, the person usually does regain some or all of the weight that was lost initially, despite the surgery.)

As Kelly talked about her lifestyle and career, it became clear that she put many hours a day into her teaching and related administrative work. I know many hard-working teachers, but few who did as much work as Kelly. When I asked her why she put in so much time, she said that, as she was single and other teachers had families to look after, it was "only fair" that she do more of the extra work than they. She also took care of her widowed mother, who was elderly, almost immobile due to arthritis, and had serious, diabetes-related health problems. Kelly often stayed over at her mom's place rather than in her own apartment. When asked about her eating style, she described a pattern of fairly well-balanced meals, rarely missed meals, and meals that were occasionally too large. She was quite certain that she had not experienced binge eating.

Diagnostic Evaluation

A) FOOD RECORDS, UNDER-REPORTING, AND CALORIMETRY

It was quite hard to reconcile Kelly's story of long-term, and moderate, though somewhat disorganized eating with her quite excessive weight. In order to know what course to take, I needed to know more about her. After a thorough medical and social history, we agreed to meet again to review her dietary control. I did something we don't normally do this early on in assessing a patient; I asked that she keep a record of what she ate for week. I emphasized that keeping a food diary was not a test. I rarely ask for a diet record, and certainly not for more than one seven-day food record, because patients experience these as punitive and intrusive. However, where the patient or her doctor isn't sure why she gains weight, such a record can be useful if properly interpreted. The key is to determine if the patient can correctly record what is taking place with food.

Kelly's record showed that her average food intake was just over 1500 calories per day—not enough food to maintain her actual weight. I concluded that either she had really restricted her food intake while keeping the record (though she said that she had not), or she was eating more than she realized or was able to record. What should we conclude from this discrepancy between her diet record and her weight? Do we assume that she was deliberately misrepresenting her food intake? Do we look for some "glandular" or hereditary factor that influences how her body uses food, or do we look for another explanation?

To determine the truth about a person's eating habits, I start with the mathematical formulae that predict calorie needs depending on the age, sex, weight, and height of the person (the Harris–Benedict equations—see Appendix 2). According to these formulae, Kelly needed to eat more than 2990 calories per day to maintain her current weight. When asked why her recorded average intake was only 1500 calories per day, Kelly said that she hadn't been deliberately "good" with her food intake when keeping this record. She honestly believed that her record accurately represented her normal eating style. To determine whether her body was burning calories abnormally (to see if she was one of those rare individuals who have a slow metabolism), I then measured her metabolic rate using a method known as Open Circuit Indirect Calorimetry (described in detail in chapter 4). This measurement showed that in order to maintain her current weight and activity level her body would need 3100 calories a day. In other words, her metabolic rate was a bit above the predicted average! Her record of what she was eating was inaccurate by roughly 1400 calories per day. Why?

It is very common (almost 48 percent of all patients) for a patient's reported food intake to be less than what should be needed to sustain his or her current weight. One of the most frequently missed problems in dealing with overweight people is their inability to recognize that they are under-reporting their food intake.

In a study I and my co-workers did, we showed that, over a one-week period, 48 percent of overweight women under-reported their food intake by an average of 526 calories per day. Fifty-two percent of the women tested were "correct reporters" and did have diet records that compared very well with what we had measured their daily energy expenditure to be. Other research has confirmed this incidence of incorrect reporting. In short, almost half of overweight people are out of

touch with what they do with food. I emphasize that these people are *not* lying; they are simply unaware of what they are
doing with food. In fact, they use food to tune out. (I will discuss the phenomenon of under-reporting in more detail later.)
Clearly, when the real issue is a lack of awareness of what is
being done with food, diet instruction and diet record keeping
will be ineffective as weight-loss strategies.

B) MOOD STATE, SLEEP ADEQUACY, AND THEIR EFFECT ON APPETITE REGULATION

In order to help Kelly, I had to find out why she was not in touch
with what she was doing with food. To do so, I had to ask a lot
of questions about her lifestyle and moods. I also administered
several psychological tests for a quantitative evaluation of mood
states such as depression. I should add, however, that such tests
can only supplement, not replace, the all-important physician's
clinical assessment of the patient's mood.

From the various tests, and interviews with Kelly, I was able
to build up the following picture. She was the eldest in her family and had been raised to look after both her siblings and her
parents—in short, to "over function." She was the family
member everyone went to, to solve problems and to make
things turn out all right. She was very good at knowing what
people expected or needed of her and felt very guilty if she
couldn't perform as expected. She was so caught up in thinking about all her duties and so poor at recognizing her own
needs that she ate without knowing how much she consumed.
She also didn't recognize what the triggers to eating were. She
didn't appreciate that her sleep was very disturbed or that she
was using food during the daytime to "wake up" and maintain
her concentration. Kelly did not acknowledge being depressed,
but did feel she was missing a personal life. She said she found
it too hard to manage all of her commitments and still have

time or energy for personal relationships. In short, she said she felt trapped but not particularly down.

It took quite some time to get Kelly to realize that, in order to help herself, she would have to negotiate a different way of dealing with people at school and at home.

Before we addressed the problem of how to modify her eating we did some further tests. One of these was a sleep study. We found that she had sleep apnea—that is, she didn't breathe adequately during sleep and needed continuous positive airways pressure (CPAP) or "supplemental air" delivered by a facemask to improve the quality of her sleep.

As we treated her for sleep apnea, she began to feel more alert and her food intake fell. She was willing to go for walks at lunchtime instead of sitting and reading or napping. Her mood also improved as she began to create some space for a social life with friends who had always been happy to have her company but whom she had previously avoided.

Treatment for Depression

Eventually, Kelly was also able to accept what she had previously denied—that she was depressed. She was no longer working so hard that her depressed feelings were masked. At this point, Kelly was treated with an antidepressant and continued on it for fifteen months. The medication helped her to overcome her feelings of guilt, anger, and anxiety at changing the relationship with her mother and siblings so that she could have a life too.

Outcome

In the second year of therapy, Kelly began to eat regular meals that she had pre-planned. The improvement in her mood and physical well-being helped her to get more in touch with her body's signals about hunger and fullness. She was more aware of what she was eating and was better able to schedule meals rather than missing them and feeling starved later on. Over a year and a half she achieved what I think is the first prerequisite for weight loss, relief of the symptoms of a wide variety of physical and emotional problems. She then became able to act differently with food and in other areas of her life. I believe her story demonstrates that the more long-term the weight problem and the more severe it is, the more detailed a medical and psychological understanding of the issues has to be. This story explains why, for many people, a diet approach alone is not going to succeed. I hope it is also clear that significant weight loss does not happen overnight!

Kelly now weighs 240 pounds and has stabilized her weight. I think she will maintain the weight loss because she has found that "critically important core issue" I mentioned in the introduction. She discovered that she had no life outside of teaching and that she wanted a relationship. She decided that life without these changes was unacceptable and was able to overcome her fears about dealing with her family members. To her surprise, her sister and mother were more willing to accommodate her than she had ever believed possible. Her childhood fears of rejection and of feeling worthless no longer governed her life. She appreciated that to be healthy there was a cost and that the "cost" was adherence to a lifestyle that would give her some balance between work and play.

Before leaving Kelly's case, we need to consider the diet teaching that she had had over the years. Kelly knew all the right answers about food intake and had been put on many diets. She would believe she was adhering to a diet, and clearly could do so for a few weeks or months. At times of added stress, however—for example, when she was overtired, or worried about her mother or school issues—she would, without realizing it, eat far more than she needed. In her case, food was a means by which she tuned out the world.

Her problem with obesity was never due to a lack of information about diets. She could recall many of them. She couldn't regulate her food intake because of other issues.

What We Can Learn from Kelly's Case

Psychological tests often show that an overweight person's "drive for thinness" (desire to be thinner) is low. It may seem surprising that a person attending a weight-loss clinic has a low drive to be thinner. In fact, however, the inability to make a push to lose weight results from a complex combination of psychological and physiological factors. When I explain this to patients, they are often relieved. Most overweight people feel that they are unable to lose weight because they have no strength of will. They see this as a sign of inadequacy. Conversely, they feel empowered when they learn that there are good reasons why they can't adhere to a diet and that they are not merely "lazy" or "weak-willed."

When an overweight person cannot succeed in losing some weight, it is almost certainly because he or she has other priorities (whether acknowledged or not) or medical/psychological problems and cannot focus adequately on food control or the need for activity. One study I am familiar with has shown that most overweight people know quite well what constitutes a healthy diet. There are many reasons why they can't eat a normal amount of food reliably, but ignorance of the correct way to eat is not usually one of them.

Some of the reasons why an overweight person may last only a couple of weeks on a diet before "falling off the wagon" are:

1. Inability to maintain a sleep pattern, work pattern, mood state, and social life that allow them to "read" signals about when they need to eat and when they have had enough.
2. Inability to distinguish sensations of hunger from feelings of anxiety, fatigue, pain, upset stomach, heartburn/nausea, loneliness, boredom, and so on. The person senses all of these feelings as hunger and eats not because of a real need for nutrients but to alleviate the fatigue, boredom, etcetera. As a result, the food is usually excess to requirements, and weight gain naturally follows.

Case 2: Binge Eating to Suppress Anger

"Mark" is a salesman in his late thirties who covers a very large territory. He buys goods that have been damaged from insurance companies and then repairs and sells them. The business is very competitive, and Mark drives hundreds of miles a day to evaluate the damaged goods on-site. He eats breakfast at 7:30 a.m. and then usually doesn't slow down to eat again until 4:00 p.m. when calls from insurance adjusters slack off. He then feels ravenously hungry. He starts eating at that point and cannot stop until he is far too full. He is of average height and weighs just over 350 pounds (158 kg).

Mark's childhood provided some clues about why he couldn't tell clients that he would call back after lunch, or, for that matter, put his car phone on a call-message system in order to eat lunch undisturbed. His reluctance to eat before he had finished the day's work was a holdover from his father's dictum that work was done before any personal pleasures, and certainly before eating. "The job comes first" was the message. Whenever Mark was perceived as slacking off, his father reacted with ridicule and emotional coldness that Mark remembered as very scary. He could not get past that training of years ago, though he understood intellectually why he needed to eat regular meals.

Mark also didn't realize that his reaction to his father's approach was to feel angry and to eat to forget the anger.

Weight-loss Background

When I first saw him, Mark had adult-onset obesity-related diabetes, severe (undiagnosed) sleep apnea, arthritis in his knees, reflux esophagitis with marked heartburn, and elevated cholesterol. Though he now knew about these medical problems, he couldn't correct his eating pattern. He had been on all the common, commercial weight-loss diets through the years and had lost weight only to regain more than he lost. Diet teaching was not necessary and, in fact, would have been very counter-productive at the start of treatment. It would have made him angry, and, as we found out later, would have exacerbated his problems with appetite control.

When Mark realized that initially he wasn't going to be given a diet, or even be weighed on his first visit, he said: "I came expecting a diet, not a lot of questions about everything but my weight. I assumed you would be another doctor who wouldn't understand that I know how I should be eating but I just can't do it."

Here is a key point to think about when seeking help with weight loss. Does the clinician or dietician see the excess weight as THE SYMPTOM of a problem or problems, or as THE PROBLEM itself? Giving you a diet to follow, plus some words of encouragement, is the "your-weight-is-the-problem" approach. This approach rarely works. In fact, the words "Let's get you started on a good diet first" simply confirm for the client, whether consciously or not, that the physician or dietician sees him in only one dimension—as a "fat person" and does not really understand why food control is poor. For many overweight people, an internal psychological barrier goes up when they are given a diet as the first step in management of their obesity. There is a brief moment of relief as their hand closes on the diet plan, but within days they feel the same old sense of not being understood or heard. This is one reason diets accompanied by behavior-modification classes often fail.

Diagnostic Evaluation

MEDICAL WORK-UP, SLEEP STUDY, PSYCHOLOGICAL EVALUATION, AND ART THERAPY

Mark had all of the assessments Kelly had and several others as well. He needed a variety of medications and had to start on supplemental air given by facemask during sleep to control sleep apnea.

As his medical care was not unique, there is no need to mention it in any detail. Once his diabetes, sleep apnea, and chronic pain from arthritis and heartburn were treated, I expected him to begin to eat in a more controlled way. That did not happen, however, and he lost only a couple of pounds. Certainly he felt much better and was encouraged to see that, with the supplemental air, he had much more energy on arising and throughout the day.

I had waited to see if Mark's ability to take better care of himself would come when he understood what it had cost him to have his father die of heart disease at only forty-eight years of age. I was sure that he understood what it meant to have obesity-related diabetes, severe sleep apnea, arthritis, and hiatus hernia at only thirty-eight. He had two sons who were his pride and joy, and he had never until now recognized that unless he took care of himself he would leave them without a father before they had grown up. So why was he not doing better with weight loss?

I had felt from the outset that he was depressed and anxious, but had waited to see if the treatment with supplemental air would help. As it hadn't, Mark was started on an antidepressant, and after several months his mood improved. However, his food intake was still high and his meals were as disorganized as ever. His weight was unchanged, and he couldn't explain why he simply didn't make any time to look after himself. He still would neglect to eat until late in the day and then binge eat in the evenings.

I asked one of our group, an art therapist colleague, Charmaine Michael, to see Mark. I did this because much of his childhood history was full of relationship problems that provoked a great deal of anger, and he was having no luck at all verbalizing the anger or understanding what to do with it. I knew that art therapy, which is very good for drawing out issues that the patient finds hard to put into words, might be ideal for Mark. Not surprisingly, his drawings showed a great deal of anger and a very poor self-concept. I was a bit taken aback, because I had not appreciated just how angry he still was even though his mood was better. Clearly Mark could hide things very well. It was through the art therapy that he began to see that his anger at a number of events in his life had blocked any further progress at helping himself. His anger was being turned inward and was very destructive. About this time, Mark saw another doctor who prescribed diet pills. Not too surprisingly, these did not help at all. (We do not see the desired effect with diet pills where someone has undiagnosed and untreated sleep apnea or a mood disorder such as depression. These drugs are also generally ineffective where eating is in response to a strongly felt emotion such as anger, rather than the result of true hunger.)

Summary

Mark still has not lost weight, but is now committed to seeing if he can work in art therapy to deal with a particular issue in his life that caused him great anger. It is important to note that it was only after I had been working with him for a year that he was able to recognize anger as a major contributor to his excessive food intake. Anger was his real issue. Another approach we have begun with Mark is cognitive behavioral therapy. Briefly, this therapy, done in writing, helps people identify how thought patterns they have grown up with are causing mood states such as anxiety, depression, and so on. For example, some people think that they are to blame when things around them go wrong. This tendency to personalize can cause anxiety and a sense of inadequacy. Once such a pattern is recognized and seen to be unhelpful, improvement can occur.

Case 3. Eating as a Consequence of a Serious Hereditary Mood Disorder

"Deborah" came to see me with a history of being unable to lose weight since her early twenties. She was a very pleasant forty-year-old scriptwriter for TV shows. At 5 feet, 5 inches (162 cm) tall, she weighed 270 pounds (122 kg). Her weight gain had been slow and steady since her late teens but had really begun after the birth of her first child. She developed what sounded like a post-partum depression that continued for some months. By the time I saw her she had lost and gained back hundreds of pounds but now found herself unable to diet any longer. The thought of going back on a diet left her feeling depressed and anxious. Not surprisingly, her health was suffering. She was worried about marked arthritis in her knees, shortness of breath on exertion, menstrual irregularities requiring ongoing medication, high blood pressure requiring several medications, and borderline diabetes.

I asked her how she currently experienced difficulty with food control. She said that her worst times were when she was feeling really good and energetic. Then, she said, her eating became impulsive and she recognized that she ate far too much. It sounded from her description as though her eating had a binge quality, as though she was "out of control" and didn't stop eating until she was far too full. However, after a binge, though she would feel a bit ill, she didn't feel guilty or upset with herself and her energy would still be high, symptoms that are atypical for most "simple" binge eaters. During the times when her eating was out of control, she needed very little sleep, perhaps only four hours a night, and was very busy writing scripts for TV shows, calling friends late at night, and so on. These periods of excess eating lasted for up to two weeks and were almost invariably followed by a period of depression when she would feel a failure, have trouble getting out of bed in the morning, and be irritable and anxious. In fact, her mood changes had got her into trouble with her employers on several occasions, since she was very unreliable about getting to the office during her down times. By this time, it was fairly clear that Deborah was suffering from a mood disturbance that had made appetite control very difficult. I asked her why she had not seen anyone about the mood problems, though she had been to a number of clinics about her weight. She said that it had not been suggested and, where she came from (in the States), mood problems were frowned on more than weight troubles, and when you were having a tough time emotionally you were supposed to sort it out yourself.

By anyone's standards she had a great work ethic, but she truly believed that her trouble with weight control stemmed from a failure to work hard enough to overcome her shortcomings. I didn't agree at all. She was relieved when I told her that I thought we needed to stabilize her mood before we could treat her weight problems. I was convinced that she had a bipolar or manic-depressive disorder, and thought her binge eating might disappear once she was on medication to reduce her mood swings. I therefore referred her to a psychiatrist who specialized in bipolar disorders.

Bipolar disorder is an inherited disease in which a person suffers from abrupt mood swings ranging from depression, accompanied by low energy, to euphoria, accompanied by high energy. There are similarities between disorders of impulse control, such as binge eating, and this mood disorder. Deborah was seen at the psychiatric clinic, and was confirmed as having bipolar disorder, a condition her mother and aunt also seemed to suffer from. She was started on Epival to moderate her mood swings. Lithium, a drug commonly prescribed for this mood disorder, was not used because of the tendency of some people to gain weight while taking it. Epival can also cause weight gain; however, within two weeks of starting her medication Deborah was feeling better than she had in years. Her eating was under much better control, she was able to lose some weight, and after a few months she had lost almost 40 pounds (18 kg). Unfortunately, her mood began to deteriorate again and she became quite depressed and began to binge eat. Her medication was then adjusted to include a Prozac-like drug known as Zoloft. This was added in a small dosage to prevent the depression from returning.

Summary

Deborah had a fairly uncommon mood problem and, because of social pressures, had not received appropriate treatment for it. When her mood swings were treated she was able to lose weight.

I began this chapter by discussing some of the symptoms both of classic eating disorders and of the rather different problem of disordered eating. Inevitably, the discussion soon turned from the symptoms to the causes of those symptoms. In most cases, I find, weight-loss efforts succeed best when the reasons for overeating are understood and the *whole* problem is treated, not just the symptoms. The next chapter describes the process of looking for reasons. It also includes a sample questionnaire that can be helpful in the diagnostic process.

2. The Search for Reasons

Diagnosing obesity is simple. Identifying the reasons for it is not. Yet these reasons need to be addressed before any weight-loss program can succeed.

The discussion of history-taking and the "diagnostic" questionnaire at the end of this chapter are useful tools for identifying troublesome areas of people's lives that may be contributing to a pattern of disordered eating and weight gain. The questions were developed over many years of observing disordered eating patterns and trying to explain and treat them. The case histories that follow give an idea of where the questions came from, as the search for understanding, and for effective treatments, unfolded. Sadly, the first case describes a failure rather than a success—a failure that made the search for answers seem particularly urgent.

The Case of Ed

People cannot be frightened into losing weight. If you are overeating for reasons of depression, stress, or eating disorder, finger-wagging warnings about health problems will not persuade you to lead a different life or enable you to change your diet. Indeed, warnings that depress or scare you may actually reduce your ability to help yourself.

"Ed" was in his early fifties and had high blood pressure, worsening angina, adult-onset diabetes, and arthritis. He was a very generous man, gave a lot of money and time to charity, and was also very personable. Ed's doctor had put him on several diets, but even if he lost a little weight he always more than regained it. When I first saw Ed he told me that he had lost some weight at a commercial center years earlier, but had regained all of it plus more and just couldn't contemplate trying that route again. Both he and his doctor were hoping I had a better way.

That was my first year of practice, and the only "new" approach I could offer was what we termed a "Protein-Sparing Modified Fast," which was essentially a diet of meat, fish, or chicken, just enough carbohydrate to prevent ketosis, and with a lot of supplemental minerals and vitamins. It had been proven safe if properly done and was great at lowering weight, blood pressure, cholesterol, and blood sugar. Ed took a look at it and said that he couldn't do it because he was so busy he would miss meals or forget to take his supplements. He had clearly come to see me only to please his doctor, not because he was personally committed to losing weight.

I fell into the trap of getting right into the weight issue with Ed rather than taking the time to discover why he had such a severe eating problem. I was worried enough by his condition that I did what everyone else did with Ed, hurried to try to help him attain some weight loss.

I thought that perhaps regular diets might work if we could get him to adhere to these by breaking the steps down into small dietary changes every few days. He tried hard, or so it seemed based on his recollection of meals, but the scale didn't show any weight loss. After about two months, his angina was getting even worse. His cardiologist started him on nitroglycerine paste applied to the skin twice daily, and he used other oral medication to lower his blood pressure. I knew Ed was depressed and didn't sleep well, but I was much more concerned about the angina. His heart disease made it unsafe for me to prescribe drugs that might have had a weight-modifying effect, and his sleep problem did not respond to mild sedatives. In retrospect, he likely had sleep apnea, but we didn't investigate that. In the early 1980s we didn't understand just how prevalent it was.

In a fit of frustration one day, I told him that if he didn't "grow up" and start acting differently—stop working so many hours, volunteering at his kids' school, coaching hockey, ignoring the need to rest or relax, and so on—he would likely die. He listened politely and then he said something I will always remember: "Doctor," he said, "even if you told me I was going to die a month from now, I don't think I could do anything differently." As it happened, his words were prophetic. He died almost exactly a month later, collapsing one morning while working in his office.

It shook me up that I hadn't seen that he was, in a way, not competent to look after himself. He had seen psychiatrists and taken psychiatric screening tests for depression but was not thought to need treatment. Nevertheless, though he was psychiatrically normal by everyday criteria, he was out of control and not in charge of his life.

Warnings about the dire consequences of his health problems did no good. Because the real reasons for his overeating and overworking were never determined and dealt with, diets and advice about behavior modification proved useless. It is a real irony that I know what I would do for him today.

If you are not doing what you know is in your best interests, ask your doctor to help you find out why. Some difficult life situations force us to develop abnormal coping mechanisms. If obesity is due to the effects of depression, bulimia, binge eating disorder, other mood problems, chronic pain, tiredness or certain gastrointestinal problems, the root causes will need to be identified and treated first or no success is possible. If Ed came to me now, I would take a very different approach. To begin with I would have sought to deal with his symptoms of poor sleep, pain, angina, binge eating disorder, and "running depression" (explained later on). I would not have addressed his diet directly. Of course, he could still refuse to cooperate, and perhaps the outcome would be the same.

The next case illustrates how long it can take to understand the complex reasons for weight problems. In "The Case of Stephanie," diagnosis and treatment evolved gradually in a process of trial and error.

The Case of Stephanie

Putting your life on hold in order to help others can produce anger and anxiety, which, in turn, can lead to overeating. "Stephanie," a bright, well-dressed, forty-year-old, came to see me with a twenty-year history of huge weight fluctuations during periods of depression. The first such episode occurred when she was eighteen and found herself eating compulsively during the Christmas holidays. She had been "dumped" by her boyfriend and was very angry and humiliated. By May, when she felt herself regaining control over her appetite, she had gained 40 pounds (18 kg), but was able to lose most of the weight. Over the years, she clearly had weight gain associated with (undiagnosed) seasonal affective disorder (SAD), but she steadfastly denied that her weight changed with emotionally charged issues. When she came to me, she weighed 340 pounds (154 kg). Her height was 5 feet, 5 inches (165 cm). She wanted to lose weight, she said, because she was worried about her health and the example she was setting for her seven-year-old daughter.

Stephanie was well educated, very accomplished in many ways, and obviously highly intelligent. It seemed odd to me that she had not sought medical help for her weight swings before now. Was she shy about asking for help in general?

There were other, more specific questions, too. Why had she gone from diet to diet only to gain back more than she had lost? Why did she not seek help for the SAD symptoms that kept her in bed half the day from December to March? Why was she seemingly unaware of how much she was eating?

Stephanie was the only child of parents who were now very elderly though still fairly healthy. The family was wealthy and prominent in the community. Stephanie's father ran a large local business that employed nearly 75 percent of the townspeople, and he had a strict family code of conduct. Asking people outside the family for help just wasn't done. As the only child, who would one day take over the business, Stephanie was taught from an early age that she had to preserve her name and reputation in the community. As a teenager, she had felt unable to go to the local doctor for help, as he was her dad's friend. Nor could she admit to her parents that she was unhappy about her weight. Her parents were silent about her weight, so she assumed they felt it was a problem she should solve on her own.

Clearly, she had grown up with a fair bit of pressure to conform to family values. In addition, she felt she was expected to keep her father's business running, though she didn't really want to. In fact, she had changed her course in life several times to accommodate her parents' needs: at one point, for example, she left her teaching career to help restructure the family business for a merger.

She acknowledged that she was frustrated and felt that her life was on hold, but didn't connect these feelings with her eating problem. She had many rationalizations to explain why what she was doing for her parents was correct. She also claimed that she didn't feel particularly depressed once out of the SAD months. We didn't begin to get somewhere until she was able to recognize that her urge to eat was triggered by anxiety and that such anxiety-related eating had an out-of-control, binge-like quality. That is, at various times and for no clear reason that she was aware of, she would find herself in the kitchen eating.

Stephanie had been seeing me for almost a year before she identified a problem with bingeing. Once she was persuaded that binge eating could be treated with medication, she agreed to try one of the two drugs proven effective in managing binge eating disorder, Prozac (the other is Zoloft), and responded for a while with good weight loss. After five months, however, the drug seemed to lose its effect. We tried other medications with the same result. Initially, she would improve on the new agent and then it would lose effectiveness and she would regain the weight once more. With medication, her moods continued to be stable during the SAD period, but even when her mood was good her eating control would periodically evaporate.

I was very puzzled. She now had reasonable mood control, and she would do her physical exercises and stick to a reasonable diet on and off. But at times she still felt compelled to overeat. Why? I suspected that the eating was masking something that occurred fairly often and that made her very angry. Unexpressed anger can create an eating style such as hers, where medication fails because anger levels rise. However, the cause of the anger remained mysterious. Finally one day, when we were talking about her plans for the next five years or so, she said she wanted to emigrate to Australia. If she could just get away from this climate and live in a warm sunny place, she felt her mood would stabilize without medication. I knew that she and her family could easily afford to move, and she had friends in Australia. Why not go now, I asked?

Because she had to wait until her parents were dead, she said. She couldn't face leaving them. They were too old and too proud to get outsiders to help keep the house up. And she was their only child. She probably couldn't go for another five or ten years. Her parents were in their late eighties, so perhaps she was overestimating their potential longevity. The point was, however, that her life was on hold.

In fact, as we looked back over her life from college to the present, we found that Stephanie had put many important life decisions on hold, either because she felt her parents would not approve or because they might lose "face" in the community. She had even spent several years doing an hour-and-a-half commute from her home to her parents' town to help run the family business, and had given up her career to do so.

I have seen patients who felt that staying obese had a positive as well as negative side. Stephanie's weight prevented people from expecting too much of her. When she achieved something special, people were pleasantly surprised, but she didn't feel pressured to perform. As well, without being aware of it, she was using food to rebel against her parents' image consciousness and indirectly express her anger at being "trapped."

After several discussions about these ideas, Stephanie could accept that there was a connection between her obesity and her parents. As she thought about it, she felt more and more anxious and unsure of what to do with herself. She had subordinated her own needs to the "greater needs" of the "family" for so long that she found thinking about her own needs very disturbing.

Stephanie is now working in art therapy and with cognitive behavioral therapy to try to reduce her anxiety. She needs to find a way to feel all right about confronting her parents about the business and her need to be free of it. I think she will find that they are far more willing to let her go than she imagines. Her fears about their being angry or disappointed in her were based on her dealings with them when she was a child and teenager and her parents were at their most forceful.

In summary, Stephanie had been suppressing her own needs and wishes for a long time. Her anger and sense of powerlessness and loss at letting others run her life were quite normal but made her feel guilty. Instead of dealing with the issues head-on, she covered them over with a binge. Family events occurred often enough that she would be getting over the eating binges just when the next family obligation came up.

Although Stephanie was taking the anti-bulimic drug Prozac, the anxiety that triggered her bingeing needed some additional control. Buspar was added to her medication, and it has stopped the binges. However, she now knows that real progress depends on her changing her behavior with her parents. An important point to make is that none of these drugs provides "bullet-proof armor" to stave off all problems. Far from it. Currently, anxiety is the emotion she is most aware of. I imagine anger and depression will come next, until she is able to create a life where more of her own needs and wishes are met.

As Stephanie's case shows, anxiety and anger arising from unresolved personal issues can be quite difficult to treat. Sometimes, however, as in "The Case of Steve," the patient's history points to a readily treatable condition as the source of the binge-triggering anxiety. In these cases, quite dramatic improvements can occur.

The Case of Steve

"Steve" was very tall at 6 feet, 6 inches (198 cm), and weighed 400 pounds (180 kg) at age thirty-four. He worked as a book-keeper and general office manager for a small company in the transportation business. His parents had started it and he had worked with them in one capacity or another since he was twelve. He had found going to school very anxiety-provoking. He recalled that he couldn't concentrate, and that the kids in his class made fun of him for his height and his frequent errors. He was briefly the class clown until his impulsivity got him into trouble. At age twelve he began to experience panic attacks about school, and as his size made it difficult for any-one to force him to attend, he was allowed to stay at the office and work. In this environment he was accepted, and there were few time limits on tasks. There was also very little scrutiny other than from a mother who was endlessly patient with him and rarely critical. He could spend as much time as he needed on a project and would be rewarded for it. Steve was very useful at different jobs, was into every facet of the busi-ness, and could spend many hours getting the accounts into perfect shape. He got some praise for this and spent long hours in the office, so much so that he took no care of himself. By the time he was in his twenties, he was able to run some aspects of the business quite well, capitalizing on his people-management skills, and letting others handle the paperwork, which he now recognized others could complete much more quickly than he could. If he could not quickly solve a problem he tended to become so anxious that he would simply put it away to be done later. More than once this procrastination got him into trouble when bills weren't paid on time. He also tended to put every bit of his energy into a piece of work, not allowing himself to eat until the job was done, even if it took all day. Steve was also very unsure of himself. He had little confidence in his own judgment, obsessed over every point, and made himself very anxious and depressed, while trying hard to hide these feelings from everyone.

When Steve came to see me, he had been unsuccessful in losing weight and now had a very unfavorable blood-cholesterol level and early adult-onset diabetes.

Steve ate when he could get himself untangled from his seemingly obsessive need to finish tasks given to him. We eventually realized that the long hours he spent on a job would not have been necessary if he had been able to do the work efficiently. Clearly, his mental concentration was very poor, although his ability to stay seated in one place was very highly developed. When he finally finished a job, he would overeat. There were also times, as he later felt safe enough to tell me, when he cruised around town stopping at fast-food outlets buying junk food to binge on in private.

Steve was also quite depressed when I saw him. He was started on Zoloft and his mood improved markedly. However, his inability to work efficiently was still a problem. He had a very poor self-image and no confidence that he could succeed in work outside the family business. Relationships with women were seen as too risky. The women he was attracted to were generally bright professional types, and he didn't think he was smart enough for them.

Steve's history suggested he might have an undiagnosed attention deficit disorder (ADD). Though he compensated as well as he could, his inability to concentrate left him underachieving and feeling very bad about himself. Psychometric testing revealed that he had bona fide ADD. Interestingly, psychiatrists who had seen him years earlier had not recognized the ADD as an antecedent to his depression and binge eating. Steve was started on Dexedrine, an amphetamine that is used in adults with this disorder. He is much better now, with an enhanced ability to deal with business problems. As he experiences success in areas he previously saw only failure in, his self-esteem is improving. He lost 35 pounds (16 kg) in the five months after starting on Dexedrine, mainly because he can now focus on planning a meal and can remember to time meals correctly so that he does not go for many hours without eating. (I want to emphasize that the weight loss was not due to the short-lived appetite suppressant effects of Dexedrine. This drug was used in the 1940s to 1960s as a diet pill but was stopped for many reasons, not the least of which was that it did not promote long-term weight loss and had harmful side effects if used in a "weight-loss" dosage. It is, however, safe if used properly in ADD.

By giving some idea of the wide range of factors that can affect people's eating habits and cause them to gain weight, these three cases suggest why identifying the reasons for weight gain is the key to treatment.

History-Taking: Questions You Should Expect to Be Asked When You Go for Help with Weight Management

To help identify as many of the potential causes of weight gain as possible, diet consultants should try to find out as much as possible about some key aspects of patients' background circumstances. They will need to take a "history" that covers the points discussed below. To help your consultant help you, you should try to be ready with answers to these questions.

When I first meet patients, even though I have a letter of refer-ral from their family doctor describing the problem, I ask "Why did you come and, in particular, why at this time?" I want to be sure that patients are not present under duress, for one thing, and that they have thought about whether the time is right for this form of endeavor. I am particularly interested to know if they have a "core reason" for wanting to address their weight problem right now. For example, teenagers who come because their parents tell them to will often not feel com-fortable talking about the problem, especially if they feel their parents are punishing them for being overweight. Similarly, a woman coming in response to her husband's loss of interest in her because she has become overweight is not ready to lose weight until this issue is dealt with.

I then ask about *family history*. I want to know if their par-ents are living, and if they have suffered from weight problems or other medical problems such as thyroid disease, diabetes, or early heart attack (a heart attack occurring in an individual less than fifty years of age). It is critical to inquire about whether parents or grandparents had problems with mood, alcohol, or drugs. I also want to know if their siblings have had any of the above problems. Genetics play a part in obesity and its causes, and a positive history of depression in the family, for example, may point to this as a cause of obesity. Then I inquire about patients' own family status—if they are married, have chil-dren, and the age and occupation or school status of each fam-ily member. I want to know how patients spend their day and how physically and emotionally challenging this is. I also want to know if family support, such as help from a parent or grand-parent, plays a role in their day-to-day life. In short, it is cru-cial to the success of any intervention for weight loss to understand patients' medical, psychological, social, and work circumstances in detail. This allows me to know which factors are affecting mood, sleep, tiredness, and so forth, and which may be associated with poor food control.

My next questions are about *sleep problems*. I need to know when a person gets into bed, how long it takes to fall asleep once the light is off, and, if it takes more than fifteen minutes, what might be causing the delay (an anxiety state, for example). It is important to understand whether there are any environmental factors, such as noisy street sounds, etcetera, that will interfere with sleep quality and whether a bed partner snores or disrupts the person's sleep. (Sometimes, too, the family cat will disturb a person's sleep, as these nocturnal animals pace around.) I need to know whether patients snore, choke, thrash, or kick during sleep (sleep apnea and nocturnal myoclonus). It is necessary to know the number of hours slept (is it less than seven?) and whether they awaken feeling rested or tired, have a headache on arising, feel dopey, or suffer from poor concentration (sleep apnea). Also, is there any time during the day when they are almost certain to feel tired? People who are tired during the day despite adequate hours of sleep may have a problem. To determine if such people are "hypersomnolent" (more tired than normal) I ask if they would be likely to fall asleep within five minutes if they were put in a dark, quiet room. Hypersomnolence is another way sleep problems announce themselves even where people do not acknowledge poor sleep. A variety of medical conditions can also cause tiredness—such as, for example, low iron stores. Low iron is often missed because the family doctor only looked at the hemoglobin ("blood count") level. It is often forgotten that hemoglobin remains normal until all iron tissue stores are virtually depleted. For a person to have full energy, and a normal mood state and level of concentration, cellular levels of iron have to be normal, and a normal hemoglobin does not guarantee this. Ferritin levels need to be measured; as well, where a person has had inflammation or illness, other measures of iron stores have to be made, since ferritin measurement can be misleading in such cases.

I then ask about *physical wellness*—what doctors call a "systems enquiry." This involves going through questions about past and present symptoms of heart or breathing problems, trouble with digestion, and gynecological problems including PMS and associated mood, appetite, and sleep changes. Problems with pain or limited mobility due to arthritis, headaches that are sufficiently bad or frequent enough to interfere with daily activities, and skin or ear-nose-throat ailments should also be identified. In short, I look for any sign of medical illness that could make eating control or the burning up of calories less than normal.

A *medication history* is next, including which drugs and vitamins are taken and if these have had a noticeable effect. It is very common to see patients who are being treated for a chronic condition such as high blood pressure, pain, thyroid disease, or depression and who are far from well but are "better" than before they were put on the medication. Where depression, pain, or thyroid disease has been suboptimally treated, the inadequacy of treatment can noticeably increase weight problems. In one very common scenario, a patient has been depressed, has had some treatment, and is better than before but still less well than "normal." The reasons for this only partial recovery are many, but the commonest is that the doctor accepts any sign of improvement as equivalent to a "return to normal" and does not further fine-tune the medication dose. It is also frequently the case that the patient doesn't want to complain if he or she is feeling better than before the drug was given. Some patients have been down long enough that they don't have a good idea of what "normal" feels like anymore. A relative who knew the person before the illness can often provide information about his or her normal levels of functioning. It is imperative for mood disorder to be fully treated to avoid relapse. That means getting the patient as close to normal as possible with medication and then using psychotherapy to enhance and complete the transformation. Thyroid problems such as hypothyroidism are not uncommon. We measure the adequacy of thyroid hormone replacement by measuring the thyroid stimulating hormone (TSH) level in the blood. TSH can give the impression that thyroid replacement has been adequate, but this is not always the case. It is beyond the scope of this book to go into the details of thyroid hormone replacement therapy. However, if a patient's energy, cold tolerance (ability to tolerate a cool environment as well as other people do), or concentration remains below par after thyroid problems have been treated, a more sophisticated evaluation may be necessary measuring hormones other than TSH.

The degree of *physical activity* experienced on a weekly basis is the next area of inquiry. What have patients done previously to keep active? What activity do they enjoy? (This is also an ideal place to inquire about peer group relationships, friendships, and so on.) It is also necessary to know if they stopped doing a favorite activity because of injury, arthritic pain, blood pressure problems, and so forth. We can almost always get a person who previously liked some activity back into it by carefully dealing with pain management, asthma, blood pressure, etcetera.

Job history is next, because it is important to determine whether the job is contributing to weight-regulation problems. Does the person enjoy the job, like his or her co-workers, and have a measure of control over his or her daily duties and areas of responsibility? Does the person commute daily and for how many hours? The level of stress has to be evaluated, because not infrequently a person will describe a job environment as "fine" when it sounds very hard or stressful to me. We all tend to become inured to "the battle" and hence are not always aware of stress that may be affecting our sleep, mood, or energy levels and thus making food control very difficult.

Long commutes are sometimes said to be helpful as they give you time to wind down, but I have rarely found a patient who commuted more than thirty minutes each way who did not suffer more stress and fatigue because of it. One patient I know got up at 4:45 a.m. every weekday, took the bus to the GO train, and spent an hour getting into Toronto. She worked from 7:30 a.m. until 3:30 p.m. and then commuted back, arriving home by about 5:30. She then shopped, got dinner ready, dealt with the children, and, once the kids were in bed, did housework. She got to bed about 11:00 p.m. This had gone on for nine years. This lady described her job as good but stressful, but said she did not feel especially tired or overburdened. Her full story is a long one, but the above description of what she thought of as "just fine" alerted me. Clearly, she did not have a good sense of how she was feeling or being affected by her workload. She looked exhausted, and her blood pressure was elevated. She acknowledged some tearyness but felt it was just silliness on her part. When I persuaded her to take two weeks off (and she took a lot of persuading), she became aware of just how tired and depressed she was. She needed medication for panic attacks and for what is sometimes termed a "running depression," which occurs when a person who works too hard to notice feelings of depression has an enforced "slowdown." This patient is now much better. She is determined that she won't let herself get run down like that again. She said afterwards that the effects of the job had happened so slowly she didn't even see the mood problems creeping up on her.

I also take a *diet history*, asking what patients have tried in the past to see if there is a particular pattern of trouble. Uncovering a pattern of response to diets in the past is important, because knowing how patients have handled earlier efforts at weight loss tells a lot about what NOT to do. For example:

1. In the first common pattern, patients report going on a commercial diet program, often with a friend, losing weight for three or four weeks, and then "falling off the wagon." It is essential to determine just why they lost interest. Most commonly, it is because the diet left them feeling deprived and one or more of the five main causes of obesity was present but not dealt with. Going ahead with dietary advice at this point will not result in weight loss.

2. In another pattern, patients lose weight over a number of months but become more and more anxious as weight loss proceeds and people begin to notice the changes. They then "panic" and go off the diet. Weight is generally regained very quickly in such people. The problem of experiencing anxiety as weight reaches a certain point is common, and the "phobic weight" problem has to be understood and solved before weight loss can be successful.

3. In the third pattern, people stick to a diet "to the letter," and lose weight for a few weeks, but then hit a plateau. They cannot get back on track and lose weight even though they make the diet more strict. The most common reason for this failure is under-reporting and lack of awareness of what they are eating.

There are other patterns, but with any of them, the key is to be clear why the effort failed. It is extremely common for patients to say that *they* failed the diet. I point out that if a large majority of people fail to take weight off and keep it off after a commercial diet, the problem logically lies with the diet methodology and not the participant!

I also enquire about current dietary habits to learn if patients know there are four food groups and to see if foods from these are present. I then want to know if regular times are set for meals and snacks. That is all one needs to know initially. Asking for detailed diet logs is a waste of time at this stage and only tells patients that the health care provider does not know that diet inadequacies are symptoms of other issues, and not the cause of weight problems per se. I then ask what they would feed a healthy child for breakfast, lunch, and dinner and which snacks are reasonable (it is very rare for overweight people not to be able to describe a normal, healthy diet, though they may not be able to follow one themselves). I want to know if binge eating occurs and under what circumstances. Finally, I ask patients if they know what tells them to eat and how they know when it is time to end a meal. With regard to recognizing hunger, most people can differentiate between a "mouth" hunger (a craving for food or a desire for a specific taste), and real or "stomach" hunger. Real hunger is usually experienced as a growling, empty feeling in the stomach area. With regard to knowing when to stop eating, the most common problem is that people stop eating when either the plate is empty or they are full. Neither is the correct way to determine when to stop the meal.

The questionnaire that follows is another useful tool for diagnostic purposes.

Questionnaire

If you answer yes to any of the following questions you may have trouble losing weight. In some cases, the relevance of the question to the issue of weight control is obvious. Where it may not be clear, I have added a brief explanation.

1. Do you miss meals?
A habit of missing meals may reduce your ability to sense adequate fullness. A person who misses breakfast will typically become increasingly preoccupied with food later in

the day, lose the ability to sense fullness correctly, and hence be prone to overeat from about 4:00 p.m. onwards.

2. Do you eat quickly?

If you do, you lose the benefit of the feedback mechanism between your stomach and your brain that is used to sense fullness. When you eat slowly, your brain has more time to sense fullness and perhaps to register signals from hormones released in the upper small intestine indicating adequate food intake. You are more likely to "be in control" if you eat slowly.

3. Is your sleep disturbed?

Tiredness will lessen your ability to regulate food intake, be active, and maintain a stable weight. Tired people frequently eat in order to lessen their sense of fatigue. They also generally accomplish less physical activity due to being tired. If you are often tired and also overweight, find out why you are sleepy.

4. Do you wake in the morning feeling less energy than you think you should?

See question 3 above. Sleep that is non-restorative predisposes you to overeating.

5. If you had to rate your overall mood, with 10 representing your best continuously experienced mood and 0 your lowest continuously experienced mood, are you less than 6-1/2 out of 10 most days of the week?

Clinical experience indicates that if you rate your mood as usually below 6-1/2 on the 0 to 10 scale, your ability to control food is less than average and you may have trouble losing weight.

6. *If you rate your level of day-to-day anxiety on a 0 to 10 scale, are you more than 5 out of 10? (A "0" indicates no worrying, a "5" means you worry a lot of the time, and a "10" means worrying is so intense you have panic attacks.)*
   If your anxiety level is above 5, you may be less able than average to regulate your food intake. Anxiety can consume a lot of energy and preoccupy you to the point where sticking to a diet is very difficult. One person in five has an anxiety disorder, and abuse of food and alcohol may occur in an attempt to lessen the anxiety.

7. *Using the same scale as above for "anxiety," is your level of irritability greater than 4 out of 10? (A "0" denotes no sense of irritability, a "5" means you are edgy or irritable much of the time, and a "10" means you are barely able to control yourself)*
   Irritability is a very unpleasant sensation. You may try to mask it with food or other agents such as alcohol.

8. *Do you experience binge eating?*
   A binge experience is defined as follows: You have an urge to eat, and eat with an out-of-control feeling. You stop only when you are painfully full, fall asleep, vomit spontaneously due to nausea, run out of food, or are interrupted. (If you answer yes to this item, please discuss this problem with your doctor.) Binge eating, whether accompanied by the rest of the bulimic symptoms or occurring on its own, is a neurological problem—that is, the binges reflect an imbalance in brain biochemistry.

9. *Can you see a direct link between eating and emotional events?*
   In other words, will stress provoke you to eat when you are

not hungry? Emotionally based eating will definitely make you consume calories that you don't need nutritionally.

10. *Do you eat a low-fat diet and feel hungry an hour after a meal?*

I believe that because the very low-fat diets that have been advocated for the past decade are unsatisfying, they are causing some of the obesity we now see. A low-fat diet will leave you hungry, and you may end up consuming more total calories than with a diet that is moderate in fat.

11. *Have you been on a commercial diet more than once in the past few years?*

The more often you have been through a diet program, the more difficulty you are likely to have in knowing whether you are eating correctly or not. Much of the weight-loss theory given to people attending weight-loss clinics is incorrect, and behavioral advice focuses attention on learning to ignore signals of hunger.

12. *Do you weigh yourself more often than once every month when you are not trying to lose weight?*

The more often you weigh yourself, the more misinformation you are likely to get about your weight. Weight fluctuates during the month, particularly for women. Reacting prematurely to perceived weight changes can result in either restrictive eating or binge eating.

13. *Do you weigh yourself more often than every two weeks when trying to lose weight?*

Frequent weighing will result in a conflict between signals of hunger and the desire to see a certain amount of weight loss. Remember that real weight loss—that is, loss of fat rather than water—occurs slowly, and the average weekly loss rate (1.0–1.5 lb./0.5–0.75 kg) is really only detectable with weighing every two weeks.

14. *Is your level of planned physical activity less than thirty minutes of walking or the equivalent in biking, swimming, aerobics, etcetera, per day?*
There is NO way to maintain a normal weight without regular physical activity. Perhaps a decade ago, a physiologist made the suggestion that exercise taken for twenty minutes three times a week was sufficient to maintain some level of fitness. While this level of activity is better than nothing and will improve muscle strength and cardiovascular functioning, I think that piece of information did everyone a disservice. It is untrue that this level of exercise is useful in weight maintenance.

15. *Do you find it difficult to differentiate between emotional feelings and physical ones? For example, is it hard for you to tell the difference between being hungry and being angry or frustrated?*
A sizable minority of overweight people are unable to differentiate between hunger and various emotional states. This lack of awareness makes it hard for them to be sure they are eating to supply needed nutrients. If you cannot distinguish true hunger from, for example, anger or frustration, you will end up eating when you don't really need food, and will gain weight.

16. **Do you experience any chronic medical problem, such as heartburn, on a daily basis? Another example would be arthritis that leaves you with stiff, sore joints every morning and soreness during day-to-day activities.**

    Chronic pain is very unpleasant. Food may be used to combat pain, and weight gain is a common result. Activity level is often lowered by pain and the expenditure of calories reduced.

17. **Have you experienced feelings of growing anxiety or even panic spells when you were dieting in the past and weight loss became noticeable?**

    A significant number of patients report feeling more and more anxious as weight loss reaches a point where people around them begin to notice and to comment. There are several common reasons for this. For example, this response can happen with clients who have been victims of assault or who are in difficult relationships where the reactivation of a sexual relationship would be unwelcome.

18. **Do you expect weight to be lost at a rate of more than a pound a week?**

    Unrealistic expectations can lead to discouragement and make it difficult for you to persevere with a weight-loss program.

19. **Do your parents or siblings have problems with any of the following: drug or alcohol abuse, an eating disorder, or a mood disorder such as depression?**

    You may be genetically predisposed to having these problems, and any of them can cause weight problems.

20. *Is there a lot of friction in your day-to-day relationships?*
Anger and frustration or a sense of powerlessness or loss
can lead to disordered eating.

21. *Are you having trouble at work with fellow employees or*
supervisors?
See question 20 above.

22. *Have you ended a relationship in the past year and still*
feel sad about it?
See question 20 above.

23. *Do you see seasonal changes in weight and mood that are*
predictable?
I have had a large number of patients with seasonal mood
changes that had been unrecognized as causing weight
problems. These "winter blues" can be severe enough to
interfere with eating behavior and activity levels. Seasonal
affective disorder (SAD) is quite common and needs medical treatment. Your doctor can determine if you are suffering from this.

24. *If you are female, do you have pre-menstrual syndrome*
(PMS) that lasts longer than two days?
The mood changes, feelings of fatigue, and increased food
cravings can lead to weight gain if they are present for long
enough.

25. *When there is a job to be done, does everyone tend to ask*
you to do it?
You may subordinate your needs in order to get the job
done and not look after yourself correctly.

26. *Are you highly regarded as a person who steps in and smooths out difficult situations? For example, do people turn to you to deal with situations where there are angry feelings?*
See question 25 above.

27. *Do your responsibilities (e.g., job, children, spouse, etcetera) leave you feeling overwhelmed?*
You may try to reduce or cope with this feeling by eating excessively.

28. *In your day-to-day dealings with people, do you often end up feeling guilty for not doing the "right thing"?*
See question 27 above.

29. *Do you know the difference between average and mediocre?*
A great deal of energy can be spent on doing tasks very well when all that was necessary was an adequate job. If you are a perfectionist who equates "average" with "mediocre," you may eat to maintain the energy necessary to do everything in an above-average way. You will also likely suffer from performance anxiety, or the fear that you can't get something done right and eat to suppress the anxious mood.

If you take this questionnaire, your answers to the questions may surprise you. That's fine. Sometimes it can be very helpful to get a new "take" on an old problem.

In another area—when trying to determine what you "should" weigh—a new approach can also be helpful. For medical reasons, this question does need to be addressed, but I have found the standard way of dealing with it counterproductive. In the next chapter, I explain why.

3. What Should You Weigh?

With a few exceptions, the patients I see do not need to be weighed frequently, and certainly not on a first visit. Yet almost the first thing a doctor or commercial weight-loss "counsellor" will do is weigh you. Is this necessary?

In my opinion, there is no good reason to weigh someone who comes in for help with obesity. Weighing someone before you have really got to know him or her is a turn-off and may be perceived as an attempt to make the person "look bad." Furthermore, weighing someone, especially on a first visit, adds nothing to the physician's understanding of why the person is overweight.

It is true that there are statistics that help to define the level of risk people face based on their degree of overweight. Patients at highest risk are those with a Body Mass Index (BMI) above 35. (Remember, the Body Mass Index is the measure used by the World Health Organization to determine levels of obesity. It is discussed more fully below.) Certain blood tests, such as those for cholesterol level or blood sugar, are also useful for assessing a person's health risk. However, for practical purposes, one can tell approximately how much overweight people are simply by looking at them. Weighing can come later, when the doctor needs data to compute Body Mass Index or some other weight statistic.

My experience is that an initial weigh-in often creates animosity, which both client and doctor may be unaware of but which may surface later on and negatively affect treatment. I therefore suggest that clients decline to be weighed if they feel at all uncomfortable about it. One of our therapists makes a point of discussing the issue with the client before any weighing is done. She finds it useful to ask what feelings the idea of being weighed causes.

Determining Correct Body Weight: What "Should" You Weigh?

Clients have different ideas about what they should weigh. Some of these ideas are counter-productive. There are different standards for "normal" weight and some of these reflect society's values. Estimating your health risk from obesity is a useful place to start. One method for doing so, developed by Jean-Pierre Despres in Quebec City, focuses on waist measurement. Despres's group determined that a waist circumference above 39 inches (100 cm) in men and above 35½ inches (90 cm) in women indicated an elevated risk of heart disease, high blood pressure, and diabetes over people who carry their excess weight around their hips and thighs. It seems that fat located on the abdomen affects how the liver reacts to insulin and processes nutrients from the diet, and also determines the rate at which the liver manufactures various substances such as triglyceride and cholesterol.

According to Despres, obesity is a serious health risk only if a person does not have metabolic fitness, which he defined as "normal values for blood pressure, blood sugar, and blood lipids [fats]." Therefore, an overweight person with normal blood pressure and normal levels of blood sugar and blood lipids is not at major risk of life-threatening illness at that point in time, and may be quite safe with relatively modest weight loss.

Here are a few ways to determine whether a person's weight is ideal or not.

1. Statistically Correct Weight: Body Mass Index (BMI)

When I ask my patients what they think is their best weight, most say that they have heard that for their height they should weigh a certain amount. This concept of correct weight for a particular height is a useful one and is used by actuaries to develop height and weight tables for life insurance companies.

It has long been recognized that there is a direct correlation between the degree to which people are above the average weight for their height and mortality. As death and illness are what life insurance is about, insurance companies spent a lot of money in the 1950s researching the connection between weight and illness. We now use a measure of weight for height known as the Body Mass Index (BMI) (your weight in kilograms divided by the square of your height expressed in centimeters). For example, to find the BMI of a man 6 feet (182 cm) tall who weighs 176 pounds (80 kg) divide 80 by 182^2, or 33 124. The result is 0.0024, expressed simply as 24. We know from actuarial records that a BMI between 20 and 24 describes a person with a low risk of obesity-related illnesses such as heart disease, high blood pressure, and diabetes.

Once BMI rises above 25—in fact, when it is between 25 and 29—we know that a person is probably overweight; if BMI is above 30, the person is probably obese.

The problem with using BMI to determine correct body weight is that for some people it will give a false report. For example, take a man who is more muscular than average. Such an individual could be 6 feet (182 cm) tall and weigh 200 pounds (91 kg) but not be overweight if the additional weight is muscle. The BMI would be 27.4, but there would be no increased risk of illness if his body fat mass were normal. Similarly, a woman could have a BMI of 23, with a weight of 132 pounds (60 kg) and a height of 5 feet, 3 inches (160 cm) and be quite chubby if she had little muscle mass and quite a bit of body fat. Her risk of ill health would be elevated even though her BMI was not high. Statistically, therefore, BMI is a good way to evaluate a large population for risk of illness, but less good for evaluating individual cases. We need to remember that statistics describe the characteristics of groups of people, not individuals.

2. Appearance in the Mirror: The "Eyeball" Estimate

Another way of determining correct body weight is simply to look at a person. Studies show that the eyeball method works quite well. In other words, people who look too chubby—or too thin, for that matter—are almost certainly outside their correct body weight.

Sometimes the person being evaluated has a distorted body image and sees herself as fat when she is not. This can be a problem if the client cannot accept another's judgment that she is normal. She may continue to feel fat despite reassurance.

3. Body Fat Measurement: The Use of Calipers and Other Measurement Techniques

Body composition (a measurement of the amount of lean body tissue—i.e., muscle—and fat the body is made up of) may be determined using skinfold calipers, and more accurate measurements may be obtained by a technique known as bio-electrical impedance analysis. Underwater weighing, ultra-sound, computed tomography (CT) scans, and radioisotope studies may also be used to determine body composition and body-fat proportions.

Table 3.1:
Percentiles for Triceps Skinfold in Millimeters (Females)

Percentile Age group (years)	5	10	25	50	75	90	95
10–10.9	7	8	10	12	17	23	27
11–11.9	7	8	10	13	18	24	28
12–12.9	8	9	11	14	18	23	27
13–13.9	8	8	12	15	21	26	30
14–14.9	9	10	13	16	21	26	28
15–15.9	8	10	12	17	21	25	32
16–16.9	10	12	15	18	22	26	31
17–17.9	10	12	13	19	24	30	37
18–18.9	10	12	15	18	22	26	30
19–24.9	10	11	14	18	24	30	34
25–34.9	10	12	16	21	27	34	37
35–44.9	12	14	18	23	29	35	38
45–54.9	12	16	20	25	30	36	40
55–64.9	12	16	20	25	31	36	38
65–74.9	12	14	18	24	29	34	36

Instructions for use of this table: Locate your age category and run across the table to find the thickness of your triceps skinfold as measured with calipers. If, for example, you are a female aged 25 to 34.9 years, and your skinfold measures 21 mm, you are on the 50th percentile for body fatness.

This means you have the average amount of body fat as determined by this measurement technique.

SOURCE: A.R. Frisancho, "New norms of upper limb fat and muscle areas for assessment of nutritional status." *American Journal of Clinical Nutrition.* Copyright 1981 American Society for Clinical Nutrition.

Calipers are inexpensive and, if used correctly in *relatively normal-weight individuals,* can accurately measure the thickness of fat at different locations on your body and allow a calculation that determines what percentage of body weight is fat (fat-fold thickness is measured at specific sites over the biceps, triceps, and subscapular and suprailiac areas). A man should be able to pinch between 0.27 and 0.47 inches (0.7–1.20 cm) of fat thickness at the mid-point of the back of the upper arm (over the triceps muscle, which can be felt along the back of the upper arm), and a woman between 0.58 and 0.86 inches (1.5–2.2 cm) in the same location. These triceps fat-fold thicknesses are the average (15th to 50th percentile for medium frame size) for men and women in their thirties and forties whose body mass index is in the range 21 to 25 (tables 3.1 and 3.2). Caliper estimations are not accurate when the Body Mass Index is over 30, although many health clubs still do these measurements and advise clients based on them.

You may encounter the other commonly used technique, bioelectrical impedance analysis (BIA), at a gym or fitness studio. This technique relies on the fact that fat contains little water and hence is a poor conductor of electricity. Lean tissues, such as muscle and internal organs, are relatively high in water content, and this intracellular water contains salts, which conduct electricity quite easily. The test is done by attaching electrodes to the wrist and foot and then sending a very low-amperage current through the body. Resistance to the flow of current is proportional to the amount of body fat. The higher the fat content, the more resistance to current flow there is. Where a person has little fat, and hence relatively high lean body mass, current flows readily. Analysis of the resistance to current flow allows a person's percentage of body fat to be calculated. It is an accurate technique if done correctly, but the large majority of gyms that measure their clients' fatness do not use the BIA equipment correctly because they do not insist on the following: a subject must not have consumed any alcohol for forty-eight hours before the test, must not have had anything to eat or drink for six hours before the test, should have emptied the bladder before the test, must not have exercised that day, and must be rested and lying flat. The test is not accurate where diuretics or laxatives are being used. For women, this test is best done around mid-cycle, and subsequent measurements should be done at the same time in the menstrual cycle so that changes in the amount of water in the body will not distort the measurement. Other methods, such as ultrasound measurement of fat thickness, underwater weighing to determine body fat, CT scans, and radioisotope dilution studies are not commonly available.

Underwater weighing has long been accepted as the "gold standard" for assessment of body composition, but the BIA measurement is nearly as good and is much easier to do if done correctly. Women need to have more body fat than men do, and for them a body-fat percentage of 28 to 32 is fine. Men should have a lower level of body fat, something in the range of 14 to 17 percent. It is important to note that too low a level of body fat is also dangerous as it can cause a variety of health problems in both men and women. For women these include problems such as osteoporosis and infertility. These are related to estrogen deficiency, and one not uncommon sign that body fat is too low is where the menstrual cycle is lost.

Table 3.2
Percentiles for Triceps Skinfold in Millimeters (Males)

Percentile Age group (years)	5	10	25	50	75	90	95
10–10.9	6	6	8	10	14	18	21
11–11.9	6	6	8	11	16	20	24
12–12.9	6	6	8	11	14	22	28
13–13.9	5	5	7	10	14	22	26
14–14.9	4	5	7	9	14	21	24
15–15.9	4	5	6	8	11	18	24
16–16.9	4	5	6	8	12	16	22
17–17.9	5	5	6	8	12	16	19
18–18.9	4	5	6	9	13	20	24
19–24.9	4	5	7	10	15	20	22
25–34.9	5	6	8	12	16	20	23
35–44.9	5	6	8	12	16	20	23
45–54.9	6	6	8	12	15	20	25
55–64.9	5	6	8	11	14	19	22
65–74.9	4	6	8	11	15	19	22

See table 3.1 for instructions for use.

SOURCE: A.R. Frisancho, "New norms of upper limb fat and muscle areas for assessment of nutritional status." *American Journal of Clinical Nutrition.* Copyright 1981 American Society for Clinical Nutrition.

I tend to avoid the whole process of determining body fat percentage with my clients. I have yet to see how this procedure benefits the client, though it is frequently offered in clinics and gyms as though it added something to the evaluation of the obesity problem. More disturbingly, I have had many female patients come in to discuss weight loss mainly because they had been told their percent body fat was too high in a health club evaluation of "fitness." These women were convinced that something was wrong with their weight. Almost without exception, they appeared to be of a healthy weight and generally had levels of body fat as a percentage of total weight in the range of 28 to 32 percent. It was hard for them to believe that healthy women are supposed to have this level of fat, but that is the truth. While skinny women may be "in" at gyms, this has nothing to do with health and may be quite dangerous to well-being in the long run.

There are several uses to measurement of body fat, such as in research studies and where it is difficult to establish correct body weight and a doctor has decided to use body fat as the determining variable. Nonetheless, most clients view these tests as degrading, and I recommend they be abandoned unless there is some point to the measurement. Body fat and fitness levels do not generally correlate, so I do not find this most common explanation of why the test is warranted particularly convincing. It is reasonable to determine if there is too much body fat around the abdomen and, if so, to look carefully at metabolic features such as the level of blood sugar and cholesterol, as these are higher where fat is deposited around the chest and anterior abdomen (apple shape as opposed to a pear shape in women). As discussed earlier, measuring waist circumference is a simple way to identify excessive abdominal fat.

4. Socially Approved Weight: The Vogue Magazine Approach to Defining Correct Weight

Unfortunately, I have some clients who feel that the size 4 to 6 models depicted in many women's magazines represent the ideal in shape and size. It is sometimes helpful to ask a patient whether the magazine layout reflects the ideal woman as seen by men or by women. Many men view these ultra-thin women as unfeminine. Women, however, usually feel that looking model-thin (emaciated) is somehow desirable and attainable despite the evidence that the average woman is a size 10. Most will accept that logically they cannot weigh less than their inherited body type allows (weight set point), but emotionally they are very reluctant to accept that all of the pictures have been airbrushed by advertising companies. Virtually no healthy woman 5 feet, 10 inches (178 cm) tall weighs 115 pounds (52 kg); this represents BMI of only 17.8. A number of studies demonstrate the impact of the media—especially advertising—on weight sensitivity in young people. Children and teens have to be helped to differentiate between an advertisement or infomercial and something that is real and fairly described.

5. The Weight at Which You Feel Best

Another measure of "ideal" weight is the weight at which a person feels strongest and most energetic. For most people who have been overweight for a long time, even a 5 to 10 percent reduction in weight makes a very big difference in how they feel and move. This degree of weight loss is also associated with a significant reduction in cardiovascular risk and the risk of diabetes. We must also be pragmatic in determining someone's ideal weight. For most people who have been overweight for a long period of time, it is unrealistic and demoralizing to aim for a weight set by the actuarial tables.

Setting Your Weight-Loss Goals

After determining the causes of overweight, our first task is to set a *realistic* goal for weight loss. I start with a medical model, since safeguarding physical health is *my* primary concern.

I suggest to clients that we should identify any risk factors for ill health and determine the amount of weight to be lost based on this. This doesn't mean that we don't encourage clients to reduce their weight towards normal (a normal BMI), but using medical criteria to establish the first target is a sensible approach. If you have a good understanding of the medical reasons for a weight goal, you are more likely to achieve it.

After we have determined whether you have a metabolic problem, we can set out a weight-loss plan to correct abnormal blood sugar levels, blood pressure, and so on. People usually find an initial weight-loss goal of 5 to 10 percent of their starting weight not too daunting a prospect. It is very important to set a goal that is achievable. Successfully losing 10 percent of your weight might encourage you to lose another 10 percent. This approach is much more constructive than starting out thinking you have to lose 100 pounds (45 kg).

In general, there is a trade-off between what a weight–height table says you should weigh and what you can realistically achieve over the next year. In my experience, most people do know what weight gives them the best compromise among appearance, strength, stamina, and freedom to live comfortably with food. Unfortunately, many overweight people have been brainwashed into believing they can achieve an unrealistically low weight and pursue that goal relentlessly: or they know on one level that they can't achieve a particular goal but cannot reconcile themselves to the fact. Such people may need their doctor's help to accept that it can be harmful to strive towards an unattainable weight goal. I remind patients that successful weight loss occurs not in isolation but in the context of improvements in other areas of life.

4. *Understanding Appetite and the Laws of Weight Loss and Weight Gain*

For many people who are overweight there are two especially annoying aspects to the problem of weight control. The first is the peculiar way in which appetite seems to work. The second is the fact that weight loss is a slow process. Understanding more about both these aspects can alleviate frustration and impatience and help you persevere when the going gets tough.

Understanding Appetite

Disordered eating—a syndrome that includes missing meals, having meals at irregular intervals, compulsive overeating, and so on—almost always leads to changes in body weight, mainly weight gain. Disordered eating is not new in terms of human history, of course. It was probably *of necessity* very common before we developed an agrarian economy where food grew on our doorstep. Prior to 11,000 years ago, we were hunter-gatherers. In those days, our ancestors didn't sit around relaxing. They hunted all day until they found food. As there was no way to preserve that food, whatever was found or killed was consumed as quickly and in as large a quantity as possible. It was impossible to predict when the next meal would be found. Days could pass without food, and these early humans developed biochemical pathways that allowed them to live off their stored body fat. To maximize body stores of energy, these early humans learned to stuff in as much food as they could whenever they found any. In short, they were adapted to starve or stuff, feast or famine.

The brain biochemistry of these early humans must have facilitated this gorging/starving behavior. I suspect that those whose brain biochemistry allowed them to excel at stuffing often lived longer than those who did not or could not "binge eat." These "expert binge eaters" were best able to survive and have offspring, passing on genes that allowed us to tolerate both fasting when food was scarce and overeating when food was abundant.

The result of this genetic legacy can be observed today. We all know people who waken "just in time" in the morning and rush to get dressed and leave for work without stopping for a full breakfast. Sometimes they eat a normal lunch—or sometimes just a small one, if they are overweight and trying to "diet." When they get home from work, they are surprised to find that they are preoccupied with food. Food thoughts take over, and they start to crave certain foods. They start to nibble and don't stop. They usually eat a full dinner, but don't feel satisfied. They often continue to eat, consuming more food than their body needs to maintain their weight. It is as if their bodies do not know that enough food has been eaten to last the night and so compels them to go on eating.

These people experience an inability to determine when they are full enough to meet their calorie needs. Quite often, people who have missed breakfast and eaten a normal or small lunch will go on nibbling all evening until bedtime. In doing so, they consume many more calories than their body needs, and these extra calories are deposited as fat. My overweight patients commonly report such a pattern.

Why does a person with this eating routine have trouble controlling food intake? To begin with, at breakfast time your body is running low on energy, and you should be addressing a calorie debt built up during the night. How big a calorie debt is there? If you eat dinner at 7:00 p.m. and finish any additional food intake by 9:00 p.m., the food eaten will be used to sustain body function overnight. Even while we are sleeping, our bodies' metabolic processes continue to burn up calories. A sleeping person will burn calories at a basal metabolic rate that is 80 to 85 percent of that used when lying quietly awake. A thirty-year-old woman 5 feet, 4 inches (162 cm) tall and weighing 121 pounds (55 kg) has a resting energy expenditure rate (number of calories per hour being burned) of 55 calories per hour. Simple arithmetic tells us that when she wakes at 7:00 a.m., she will have used up 550 calories of energy during the overnight fast. By the time she is up and dressed and on her way to work her energy expenditure will have risen to perhaps 80 calories per hour. By 12:00 noon, she has used up another 400 calories, so that her total energy expenditure since the night before is almost 1000 calories. At this point, there are changes in brain biochemistry due to the lack of nutrients, and her appetite center is beginning to set her up for disorganized eating later in the day. Suppose she eats a bowl of soup, with crackers, for lunch, for a total of 250 calories. She is still running a *deficit* of energy. She has a 1000-calorie deficit before lunch and, after her 250-calorie lunch, still has a 750-calorie deficit.

Building up a big calorie deficit causes a problem with appetite regulation. At 6:00 p.m. when our subject gets home, her calorie deficit has increased by an additional 480 calories. She sits down to dinner with a twenty-one-hour deficit of more than 1200 calories. At this point, the likelihood that she will eat in a controlled way is very small. The price of running a large deficit of calories during the day is a growing preoccupation with food and overeating when food becomes readily available. Because of our genetic heritage, when food becomes available again after a period of deprivation we are programmed for *weight gain in preference to weight maintenance*. In short, it is almost inevitable that a person who misses meals, especially breakfast, will have poor appetite control. In my experience, eating regularly throughout the day, which means planned meals and one mid-afternoon snack, is the only way to protect oneself against weight gain. By keeping up with calorie needs during the day, patients report much less overeating.

Understanding the Laws Governing Weight Loss and Weight Gain

How often have you read an advertisement stating that it is possible to lose "ten pounds in ten days" on a particular diet? That is an outright lie because it is impossible to lose that much real weight, i.e., body fat and other tissues, in ten days. Unfortunately, there are no laws that require a diet plan to be factual or safe. If losing 10 pounds (4.5 kg) in ten days was as easy as some diet plans suggest, there would be no need for anyone to write books on weight loss.

To understand the processes of weight gain and weight loss we have to know a bit about body composition and weight and how these are altered by food intake.

Our bodies are made up of water, fat, protein, carbohydrate, and minerals (such as those forming bone). When we say that a person weighs 132 pounds (60 kg) we are saying simply that gravity pulls on them with that amount of force. To create new body tissue we need the raw materials for building those tissues. For example, protein is used in building muscle. Once we acquire the protein by eating food, our body has to assemble the protein into a muscle structure. There is a "cost" of building this new tissue; that is, making new muscle requires calories of excess energy. 0.03 ounces (1 g) of new tissue might require 6 to 8 calories of excess energy. To gain weight excess calories are needed, that is calories over and above those necessary to maintain the body at its present weight.

To understand weight gain, we can use an example to show the mechanics of it. Take as an example a thirty-year-old woman 5 feet, 4 inches (162 cm) tall and weighing 121 pounds (55 kg). We know from a table of energy requirements (making some assumptions about activity levels), (the Harris-Benedict equations) that if she is very sedentary she needs approximately 1800–2000 calories daily to maintain that weight. However, for three days over a long weekend, she was out of town and ate more than usual, consuming 2300 calories daily. Thus, she overate by perhaps 300 calories a day if her activity level did not change. If it takes 6–8 calories of energy to make a gram (0.03 oz.) of new body tissue, this woman would have created $300 \div 6 = 50$ grams (1.66 oz.) of new tissue daily or 116 grams (3.9 oz.) of "real" weight over the long weekend. I use the term "real" because if our subject got on a scale and weighed herself she might see that her weight had risen by between 1.1 and 2.2 pounds (0.5–1.0 kg). This is because, when we overeat, we may retain a little extra salt and water for several days. Often clients come in worried that they have gained 2 or more pounds (1 kg) in a weekend. They need to be reassured that the laws of physics don't allow for "real" weight gain that rapidly.

The same rules apply to weight loss as to weight gain. The laws of physics don't change for anyone. This is one of the hardest facts to get across to clients. In order to lose weight you have to burn more calories than you eat.

Take as another example a thirty-year-old man 6 feet (182 cm) tall and weighing 250 pounds (113 kg). To maintain this weight he must eat not less than 3400 calories per day assuming he is not very active. If he wishes to lose weight, he must create a deficit of calories. In other words, the number of calories eaten must be less than the number burned off. If he diets and as a result consumes 1800 calories a day, he has a daily deficit of 1600 calories. Because mass and energy are interchangeable, as calories are burned off, the amount of body tissue (weight) that those stored calories come from must disappear as well. The number of calories representing 1 pound (0.454 kg) of weight is often quoted as 3500. This means that if our male subject has a calorie deficit of 1600 calories daily, in just over two days he will lose 1 pound (2 days x 1600 calories/day = 3200 calories). *I should point out that this degree of under-eating cannot be sustained for any length of time.*

Most people trying to lose weight hate the fact that weight loss is slow. If an average-sized woman reduces her intake by 20 percent—say, 400 calories per day—it will take her roughly nine days to accumulate a calorie deficit of roughly 3500, which represents a loss of 1 pound. Clearly, it takes time to lose weight. Losing 30 to 50 pounds (13–22 kg) could take a full year. If this sounds slow, consider that in studies using a combination of diet, activity programs, behavior modification, and diet pills, the average overweight person lowered food intake by approximately 6 percent over a full year of treatment. This resulted in weight loss on average of 10 percent of starting body weight (perhaps 25 pounds [11 kg]).

The most difficult clients to treat are those who believe

that getting professional help is a guarantee of rapid weight loss. Many patients are not happy with a slow and steady rate of weight loss and may be tempted to try various fad diets. To prevent discouragement—and faddism—it is important to discuss weight-loss goals (as opposed to fantasies) with the patient before we begin. Once the physics of weight change are explained, patients have the tools to understand why they need to change certain elements of their diet or activity and are better at adhering to their altered eating and exercise patterns. A well-informed patient does much better at weight loss.

The Dangers of Crash Diets

Sometimes, in spite of careful preparation, clients become impatient with the slow pace of weight loss and go on crash diets. There are several weight-loss systems that promise rapid results. However, clients who are losing more than 2.2 pounds (1 kg) a week are going too quickly. Very drastic diets may produce more rapid weight loss in the first few weeks because of changes in body-water balance (dehydration), but the rate will ultimately slow down (plateau) and you will lose much-needed muscle tissue as well as water and excess body fat. Clients say that they are doing these diets for a couple of weeks only, perhaps to get ready for a party, and that therefore they can suffer no real harm. I don't agree. During weight loss it is important to allow changes in body composition to occur fairly slowly and to try to preserve muscle mass by combining a well-balanced diet with exercise.

Forays into fad dieting can result in weight instability that leads to weight *gain* later on. Why is this? With restrictive diets, especially where the calorie intake is low enough to be more than 500 calories below daily requirement for weight maintenance (for example, less than 1700 calories per day for a fifty-year-old woman weighing 170 pounds [77 kg] and 5 feet, 4 inches [162 cm] tall), valuable muscle tissue is used up to provide fuel energy to keep body processes going. The loss of muscle tissue reduces the rate at which energy (and fat) is burned (metabolic rate) and makes it more likely that the weight will be gained back later on. Crash diets have other bad side effects, as well. Gall bladder disease is very common where a person has lost weight rapidly and repeatedly over time. Cold intolerance, hair loss, constipation, headaches, depression, fainting, irritability, and many other problems occur where diets are too restricted. More serious side effects, such as heart-rhythm disturbances, loss of bone mass, vitamin deficiency, and brain shrinkage have all occurred where severely calorie-restricted diets were used.

The type of tissue lost during weight change has an impact on long-term weight maintenance. When we gain or lose weight, the type of tissue that is added to or removed from our bodies varies depending on many factors, including our genetic make-up, the type of diet, and whether we are physically active. The rate at which we change weight also affects the type of tissue lost or gained: with very rapid weight gain, the added weight is usually mostly fat tissue, but with very rapid weight loss a significant amount of muscle as well as fat may be lost, especially if the diet is too severe or badly composed. When we lose lean body tissue, such as muscle, however, we are losing the very tissue that is most responsible for sustaining our metabolic rate. A cycle of weight gain/weight loss/weight gain causes a progressively higher body-fat content and lower muscle content. The less lean body tissue (muscle) on a person's body, the lower the ability to burn calories. This is one of the reasons why yo-yo dieting, with its rapid weight gain and loss, can cause changes in body composition over the long term

that actually make weight gain more and more likely to occur.
The bottom line in all of this is, avoid crash diets.

Calorimetry: The Measurement of Resting Energy Expenditure

In chapter 1, I mentioned that almost half of all clients with
longstanding weight problems substantially and unknowingly
under-report their food intake. The problem for people in this
group is significant lack of awareness of what they are doing
with food. For such people diet instruction and menu planning
alone are pointless.

When clients have been unsuccessful with weight loss for a
long time, I require them to have calorimetry done and to
record their food intake over a seven-day period. This is necessary to determine with certainty whether they have an accurate awareness of their food intake. If they do not, they need
to know it, and so do we. It is pointless to attempt to modify
behavior with food if the person is unconvinced that he or she
tunes out or dissociates when eating. Behavior change requires
the active cooperation of the client, and it is here that the commercial weight-loss programs fail. They cannot identify clients
who have this problem.

Helping people to deal with the fact that they under-report
is tough. Most believe that while they may not eat correctly,
they *are* aware of what they are doing.

I saw one extraordinary example of under-reporting on a
U.S. TV show. A woman was being interviewed in hospital
where she was admitted for treatment of a skin infection. She
was asked how she got to a weight of 640 pounds (290 kg).
She replied that she must have had a "metabolic problem"
because she had little money, and, on food stamps, didn't have

the cash to go out and eat large quantities of food. The host of the show and the audience seemed to find this explanation plausible. I would have said, however, that she had a serious and unrecognized problem with food control. She was probably unaware of just how much she was eating. As long as people believe they are being betrayed by their "metabolism," and are helpless to change anything, they will not be able to lose weight. With such people, calorimetry is an invaluable tool in the necessary process of re-education.

The Methodology of Calorimetry

The test is done after an overnight fast, while the client is lying down and resting. It involves measuring the oxygen consumed by the client and the carbon dioxide he or she breathes out over a period of about forty-five minutes. To accomplish this, a calorimetry machine is used.

The machine contains a carbon-dioxide analyzer and an oxygen analyzer. A hood is placed over the head of the client. Air is circulated through the hood, and the machine very precisely measures the amount of oxygen used and the amount of carbon dioxide produced as the subject breathes quietly at rest. Early in this century, physiologists learned that there was a direct relationship between the rate at which a person's cells consume oxygen and make carbon dioxide and their use of calories of energy. In other words, if a patient uses 100 units of oxygen and breathes out 80 units of carbon dioxide while in the fasted and resting state, we can calculate the precise number of calories that he or she burned. We can then determine the number of calories a day the person must eat to maintain his or her weight, allowing for activity level (see Chapter 8, table 8.1). When we compare the calories recorded on the diet record with what we know is the person's actual calorie need for weight maintenance, we can see if there is a discrepancy. As I mentioned earlier, for almost half of our clients, a one-week diet record shows a food intake at least 525 calories per day below what they need to maintain their current weight.

When dealing with a weight problem that is severe or of long duration, it is best to measure a person's unique metabolic requirement. Doing so helps the client and the doctor to understand the causes of the weight problem. If the problem is with food-intake recognition, addressing it directly will be more constructive than simply prescribing yet another diet.

Insight into these two common weight-loss conundrums—the role of appetite in disordered eating and the slow pace of weight loss—can be useful in helping you persist with your own attempts to alter your approach to food. However, before getting into any specific recommendations, I want to explore in more detail what we know about the role of the brain in appetite regulation.

5. Food and Your Brain: A Delicate Interaction

When asked how they regulate their food intake, clients say that they eat for many reasons besides hunger. Some people eat because they are tired, although they may not realize that they are eating to get the energy boost that food provides. Others eat when they are under stress, because on some level they feel that food helps them relax or comforts them.

Recent studies show just how complicated food-control mechanisms are. One of the pioneers in appetite regulation, Dr. G. Harvey Anderson, professor of nutritional sciences at the University of Toronto, showed years ago that serotonin, a brain neurotransmitter, was essential in appetite regulation. He used specially bred rats and other mammals to show that appetite regulation is the result of collaboration between several elements of the brain acting on hormonal and neurological messages from the body. As well, receptors in the brain and various other organs are sensitive to the levels of nutrients (sugar, amino acids, and fats) that cells are exposed to and even the speed with which they are using up fuel. Signals based on this information are fed to the appetite area of a person's brain and are registered as sensations of hunger or fullness.

Feelings of hunger and the urge to eat are the result of complex signals from the brain and the rest of the body. Several times a day, specific sets of central and peripheral signals determine when meals are started and how long they last. These signals include:

- messages sent along nerves from the body to the brain about such things as body temperature, stomach fullness, and exercise;
- a message from cell receptors about the level of fuel, such as glucose, that is available to cells;
- messages from body cells to the brain reporting the rate at which they are using up energy stores including fatty acids and adenosine triphosphate (ATP), a high-energy compound made by cells to store energy;
- the insulin concentration in the blood;
- the level of leptin (also known as Ob protein) in the blood (leptin, a protein made in fat cells, is released into the blood stream when fat cells are receiving food. It lets the brain know whether energy stores are adequate. It is high after a meal and low before a meal);
- the level of neuropeptide Y and other neuropeptides in the brain (neuropeptides are protein molecules with specific shapes that attach to cell membranes and cause those cells to act in various ways).

What does all this mean in ordinary language? Thirty years ago it was recognized that if a rat was exposed to cold it used up extra calories to keep itself warm and hence ate more food. If the rat was exercised it also ate more, and if it was deprived of food for a time it would overfeed itself for several days after the food restriction was lifted to overcompensate (gain more than the weight originally lost) for the weight it lost during its fast. All of these tests showed that the prime determinant of food intake is the need to achieve energy balance. In other words, the brain signals us to increase or decrease food intake in response to the rate at which energy is being used up. All metabolic energy comes from fat, protein, and carbohydrate in the diet, and experiments have been done to see which of these is used by the brain in its regulation of food.

The following brief description indicates just what these metabolic fuels do in the body.

Glucose: It was thought initially that because glucose is the preferred fuel of the brain and all nerve tissue, the level of glucose in the blood would determine appetite and food choice. However, scientific observation has revealed that while low blood sugar may trigger hunger in some circumstances and elevated blood sugar may suppress appetite, these effects are very inconsistent. We now know that glucose certainly does not act alone to modify appetite; insulin levels in blood feeding the brain are very important as well. Another way of looking at the role of sugar in appetite control was to see if there were sugar/glucose receptors in various organs that could monitor glucose levels, report the results to the brain, and trigger a change in appetite. Studies showed that liver receptors for glucose could send a message to the brain via the vagus nerve, but this alone did not account for or explain complex changes in appetite. It is more likely that carbohydrate acts in appetite regulation by affecting insulin levels and the rate at which serotonin and other neurotransmitters are made in the brain. This mechanism is not completely understood at this time. However, when clients say that they eat in the afternoon because they must have "low blood sugar," this is rarely found to be the correct explanation.

Fat: Because body fat is the major storage form of energy in the body, it has been assumed that changes in body-fat levels or in the rate of consumption of stored fat could affect food use. Although it is still felt that there is a direct link between fat levels and appetite regulation, the way in which the link operates is unclear. We do know that energy-containing compounds in the bloodstream, known as fat metabolites (e.g., free fatty acids, glycerol, triglyceride, and ketone bodies) fluctuate with the time of day (circadian rhythm) and certainly with meals. These energy-containing compounds also affect insulin release and the action of insulin on fat cells. A recent finding, announced two years ago, is definite evidence in genetically obese rats that fat cells lack the ability to make leptin. The absence of leptin seems to prevent fat cells from signaling the brain that there are sufficient energy (fat) stores and that food intake should stop. Animals lacking this substance eat too much and become obese. This leptin signaling system does exist in humans, though the way it works in obese people is very variable. It is likely that some obese people have poorly functioning brain receptors for leptin. Thus, their brains do not sense that fat/energy stores are full and that eating should stop. Others have fat cells that make less leptin after a meal than they should. However, most overweight people, probably the great majority, have normal leptin levels and, presumably, normal receptors, yet are still unable to control food intake adequately. We must conclude that leptin is not the whole story in appetite regulation and that many other chemical messengers must be operating.

Overall, it is certain that the amount of fat stored in the body plays a role in determining how appetite responds to changes in energy balance. Moreover, although the precise role of fat is not known, it is clear clinically that fat-free or very low-fat diets may lack the ability to create satiety and can leave a person feeling hungry even after he or she has eaten food containing sufficient calories. One reason I believe we are fatter today than a decade ago is the attempt to use very low-fat diets to control obesity. Such diets leave people feeling hungry. They then eat more low-fat food until they feel full. They may end up eating more calories in total than if their food had contained moderate amounts of fat.

Table 5.1:
Amino Acids: The "Building Blocks" from Which All Proteins Are Made

Essential Amino Acids*		Non-Essential Amino Acids
arginine	methionine	alanine
histidine	phenylalanine	aspartic acid
isoleucine	threonine	glutamic acid
leucine	tryptophan	glutamine
lysine	valine	glycine
		serine tyrosine

*Essential amino acids cannot be made in the body from other compounds. Thus the essential amino acids have to be obtained from foods in the diet.

Non-essential amino acids can be made from other chemical compounds already in the body.

Protein (amino acids): When a food containing protein—chicken, for example—is eaten, the intestine produces digestive juices that break down the protein into its constituent amino acids. Amino acids are the chemical molecules that are the building blocks of protein (table 5.1). They are essential for making new tissue and repairing existing tissues. They are also needed for the manufacture of enzymes, which are protein molecules that speed up chemical reactions, and for the creation of several chemicals that exist within brain cells and which are used as transmitter or messenger substances. These neurotransmitters are used by brain cells to communicate with each other. Even quite small changes in amino-acid levels in the bloodstream can affect the way the appetite centers of the brain work by affecting the levels of brain-cell neurotransmitters.

In the 1950s it was observed that food intake in humans could be increased or decreased by giving a diet that was high in protein or in specific amino acids. More recent experiments showed that giving human subjects a specific amino-acid cocktail before meals could reduce appetite appreciably. It has also been shown that a diet that is very low in certain amino acids can cause mood changes, including depression. These effects happen because amino acids change the way brain cells react and signal to one another. However, diets designed to modify amino acid levels (low carbohydrate–high protein diets) only very rarely are successful in causing long-term weight loss. Similarly, diets high in carbohydrates also fail. Changing specific blood-nutrient levels is too simplistic a way to deal with appetite regulation.

We now assume that a variety of mechanisms using sugar, fat, and protein blood levels, and signals from various body tissues, hormones, and neurotransmitters exist to regulate energy intake. The likeliest theory is that the brain initiates feeding when it gets a message from its own cells and the cells of the body that their use of fuel is beginning to fall off due to a lower blood level of nutrients. However, we still don't know how the brain receives this signal or whether particular foods can be used therapeutically to cause the appetite center to regulate food intake adequately. The brain also responds to fluctuations in blood-nutrient (energy) levels by changing the rate at which the body generates heat (the process known as thermogenesis). The more food energy is diverted to make heat, the less it is available to be stored as fat.

Food Preferences and Obesity

Even if we assume that the brain will adequately regulate total energy intake, we still need to ask ourselves how and why we prefer certain foods to others. For example, we know that people are especially likely to select carbohydrate-containing foods rather than high-protein foods in the morning. Many people choose foods high in fat and protein at dinner time, presumably because our bodies are preparing for an overnight fast. Many animals have a similar ability to select nutrients preferentially under various conditions. For example, rats will keep their intake of protein constant while increasing their total energy intake to meet exercise requirements if they are given free access to separate containers of fat, protein, and carbohydrate.

The mechanisms that control food intake in animals, including humans, are complex. Sense data related to taste, smell, texture, and appearance influence eating behavior. Energy use and storage also signal the brain to affect food intake. Finally, specialized chemoreceptors in various sites throughout the gastrointestinal tract sense the presence of macronutrients such as fat and send messages to areas of the brain that control eating behavior.

Obesity results when various factors interfere with the functioning of this very complex system. One hopeful note is the discovery that certain neurotransmitters will affect cravings for certain foods and help control appetite. Serotonin is one such neurotransmitter. It has been observed that small amounts of drugs that increase serotonin levels in the brain (e.g., fluoxetine [Prozac]) or act as serotonin-like agents (e.g., dexfenfluramine) have an appetite-suppressant effect and reduce the desire for carbohydrates relative to protein in the next meal. Another neurotransmitter is norepinephrine. Experimental injection of this substance into the hypothalamic area of the brain will increase carbohydrate desire in rats. Yet another agent, the drug amphetamine, acts on dopamine receptors, reducing total food intake, with a greater effect on protein than on carbohydrate.

The brain's use of neurotransmitters to operate a very complex system of appetite regulation is a mystery that is only starting to be understood.

Neurotransmitters, and Why Timing Meals and Snacks to Avoid Hunger Is Important to Weight Loss

Clients who want to lose weight often have difficulty accepting the importance of eating regularly during the day, beginning with breakfast. Many women say that they haven't eaten breakfast for years and if they try to they feel nauseated. Others say that when they eat breakfast they feel hungrier during the day and are more likely to overeat and gain weight. Still others claim that they don't have time to eat breakfast and don't see the connection between eating it and losing weight.

My first answer to all these objections is that eating produces changes in brain chemistry that are essential to maintaining control over food intake. Here is a clinician's explanation of why.

Assume that you have dinner between 6:00 and 8:00 p.m. About half an hour after you start eating, breakdown products from the food begin to enter your bloodstream. Over the next two hours blood-nutrient levels are rising, and by about three hours after the end of the meal they have peaked. As we sleep, nutrient levels in the bloodstream fall as they are taken up into body cells to provide fuel for metabolic actions. Some time in the early morning, sensors within the brain and in the body's cells probably identify the rate of fall-off in blood-nutrient levels. In lay terms, the brain then "forecasts" that if food is not eaten by perhaps 8:00 a.m., blood-nutrient levels will fall below the point where optimal function of all body systems is possible. Therefore, beginning early in the morning, certainly by the time most of us waken, a signal is sent to our consciousness saying, in effect, "go get some breakfast." If that signal is not obeyed, blood-nutrient levels go on falling. Activity level picks up once we are out of bed, and the rate at which blood sugar and other nutrients are used up increases. At a certain point, perhaps by 10:00 or 11:00 a.m., the brain and body cells determine that blood-nutrient levels are approaching the point where optimal functioning is not possible. As no food is coming in, some other nutrient source must be found to maintain levels of activity and brain function. The brain then decides to activate a system that allows the body to use its own stored nutrients. Certain hormones are then released that direct fat cells to liberate stored fat into the bloodstream. This fat, or triglyceride, serves as a fuel for almost all body cells. The liver is "instructed" hormonally to make sugar from its own stored glycogen and from a variety of raw materials taken from body cells. For example, muscle cells will release some of their internal protein into the bloodstream where it is carried to the liver and made into sugar. By 11:00 a.m. the process is complete and blood-nutrient levels are high enough for a person to function normally and not even feel hungry. We have all had the experience of waiting for hunger to go away and are aware that, if you simply wait long enough, the hunger feelings do actually vanish. They may do so in part because the body has made nutrients from its own cells.

Once we are "living off our own fat," so to speak, we can survive quite well for weeks if water and vitamins are supplied.

Like our prehistoric ancestors, we have the ability to stay alive even during periods of famine because we have safety systems built into our genetic make-up. If we look at what happens next, the hormones that have allowed us to draw on stored body tissue also affect the area of the brain that controls appetite regulation. The result is very predictable, and everyone who has forgotten breakfast will probably recognize what happens next:

1. We become increasingly preoccupied with thoughts of food from mid-afternoon onwards.
2. We lose our ability to sense when we are comfortably full, and to stop eating before we are in fact stuffed.

These two changes in awareness translate into changes in appetite regulation that might play out as follows. Though you eat a good-sized dinner, you are still hungry an hour later. Even if you eat again, you feel the need to keep returning to the kitchen to graze throughout the evening. Ultimately, the calories eaten at dinner and during the evening are greater than those that would have been eaten at breakfast. In other words, skipping breakfast sets the stage for overeating later in the day.

This inability to control eating later in the day is an almost universal response to having insufficient food early in the day. Once the body is forced to burn its own fuel when it is necessary to be alert and functional, subsequent overeating is inevitable. This response, which is "hard wired" into us, may have served our ancestors well, but it is making us fat. The one sure way to help people gain control over their eating is to make it possible for them to eat a breakfast that contains roughly 20 percent of the calories they need for the day.

I have never read a study detailing why a significant number of overweight people, mainly women, have feelings of nausea after eating breakfast. It may be due to an excess of gastric acid, which may reflux into the throat causing esophageal irritation. Or, increased stomach acid may be causing chronic irritation in the stomach lining. When the stomach is irritated, its emptying rate slows and nausea can be felt.

Some people say that they feel anxiety as they get ready for the day to come. Certainly anxiety is not conducive to comfortable eating and may lead to a slowing of the rate at which the stomach empties. These worriers don't feel the comfort of eating breakfast, just the discomfort of feeling bloated or that the food "just lies there" in their stomach. Irritable bowel syndrome (IBS) is another common problem that may cause discomfort and discourage people from eating breakfast (see below). It is important to try to resolve these problems rather than simply exhorting a patient to eat breakfast. People will not eat breakfast if they feel uncomfortable afterwards.

Last but not least, what about the common complaint, "If I eat breakfast, I will overeat during the rest of the day"? I would say that this is one of the most common comments I hear from my female patients.

My response is twofold. First, I explain that while it is true that eating breakfast will make you feel hunger (actually be more aware of hunger) more frequently during the day, you will also begin to feel full sooner during a meal, and will consume fewer calories over the course of the day. The result will be better appetite control and a reduction in food intake. Clients who have trouble believing this are often those who cannot recognize hunger and fullness signals equally well. They recognize a number of sensations that they call hunger very easily, but they do not recognize "full" feelings nearly as quickly. Hence, their fear that they will eat too much during the day if they start with breakfast is an appropriate one.

The second part of my response is to explain that it takes about three weeks of eating correctly, beginning with breakfast, to reawaken your appetite-control center. With many of the people I see, the recommendation to eat a meal or snack at least every four hours eventually results in much improved appetite awareness and control.

Irritable Bowel Syndrome (IBS)

IBS is a benign condition in which the bowel, principally the colon, fails to contract and relax normally—that is, the rhythm and rate of contractile (peristaltic) waves is affected.

IBS is *only diagnosed* after a doctor has ruled out other conditions affecting the bowel by doing a series of tests.

Symptoms:

- pain that is often crampy and can be severe
- constipation that can alternate with episodes of diarrhea
- gas and bloating
- nausea
- heartburn with reflux

IBS symptoms come and go. In some people stress makes these worse but there is no uniform group of characteristics to define who will be affected.

6. Essential First Steps: Dealing with Medical Conditions

Overeating often stems from the same group of fundamental problems that lead to the misuse of alcohol, tobacco, and other stimulants and narcotics. People who suffer from depression, anxiety, chronic fatigue, physical pain, or other problems may turn to substance abuse to relieve their distress. Since eating and drinking are socially acceptable, and both alcohol and food are readily available, it is not hard for someone to fall into the trap of using these for temporary relief from a mood state or physical discomfort. Alcohol causes a temporary improvement in mood, and nicotine definitely has an antidepressant effect. For most people, the association of food with comfort has been formed in infancy. The key to dealing with a dependence on such substances is to treat the mood state, pain syndrome, fatigue, or other problem.

It is pointless for a doctor to tell people to give up food, or alcohol, or anything else that is helping them cope, without offering a replacement. When narcotic withdrawal is desired, it is common medical practice to assist the withdrawal with various medications. The same is true for alcohol, where valium, Naltraxone (a narcotic receptor blocker), or similar drugs can be used to alleviate the withdrawal symptoms. However, when food intake is to be curtailed, it is exceptionally rare for the patient to be offered help in dealing with the problems that cause overeating, apart from the advice to "change your lifestyle and get more exercise." Why do so few dieticians, doctors, or weight-loss clinics consider the "side effects" of food withdrawal? I suggest it is because there is a bias against overweight people or those who binge, because they are thought to have a problem with character or willpower and simply need to toughen up. My experience is that people who overeat or drink often have a highly developed sense of responsibility, unlike some others, perhaps, who will drop a burden before it becomes oppressive enough to affect their use of food or alcohol. To encourage and help people to reduce their food intake where medically necessary or advisable, various interventions should be put in place in advance. Mood problems, chronic tiredness, pain, and so forth, should be treated *before* the attempt to deal with eating issues.

Very often, the overweight people I see suffer from one or more of the following:
- gastrointestinal problems
- chronic tiredness
- fibromyalgia syndrome
- mood disorders
- chronic pain
- binge eating disorder

In many cases, medical solutions are available for conditions such as these, and people can make significant progress with weight loss once they have addressed the problems.

1. Gastrointestinal Problems

One of the medical problems making appetite regulation difficult involves the gastrointestinal tract—that is, it involves the
esophagus, stomach, or bowel (figure 6.1). One example is
heartburn. The pain of heartburn is felt just behind the breast-
bone and may be due to the presence of stomach acid washing
up into the esophagus. If the lining of the esophagus is sub-
jected to repeated baths in stomach acid, it eventually becomes
reddened and sore. Thirty percent of people have reflux of
stomach acid by age thirty, and 60 percent by age sixty, and it
seems likely that the chronic heartburn (heartburn that occurs
more than twice a week) and stomach discomfort affect eating
regulation. In my experience, people who suffer from a
"queasy stomach" (a feeling of mild burning over the stomach,
intermittent nausea, some heartburn, and an often bloated,
uncomfortable sensation) have difficulty knowing when to eat
and how much.

The majority of patients find to their surprise that they feel
hungry less often once their gastritis or esophagitis is medically
treated. This suggests that some people are eating in response
to a feeling that they have learned to interpret as hunger but
which in fact is caused by irritation of the esophagus and stomach. *Before being treated, they ate to alleviate their feelings of
nausea, heartburn,* and so on. Cimetidine is a drug which, by
acting on the stomach cells that produce acid, reduces stomach
acid production. Recent studies show that people who have
heartburn and who are medicated with cimetidine or similar
medication lose weight more readily than those not taking the
drug. There are also many over-the-counter acid "blockers"
(non-prescription agents such as Pepcid or Zantac) that can be
helpful once a diagnosis is made. It is important to tell your
doctor about any symptoms of gastrointestinal problems you

Figure 6.1: Diagram of the Digestive System

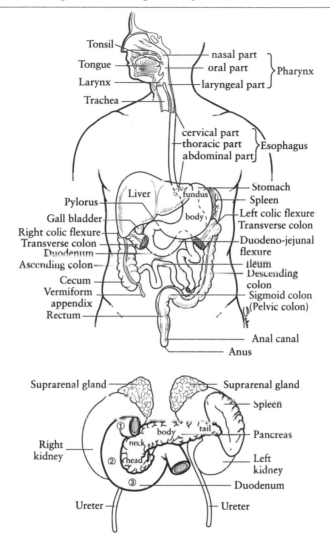

SOURCE: J.C.B. Grant, *An Atlas of Anatomy*, 6th ed. (Baltimore: Williams and Wilkins Co., 1973).

may have. Many people have felt heartburn or other discomfort for so long that they forget to mention it.

2. Chronic Tiredness

A second medical problem interfering with food intake control is that of chronic tiredness. It has been known for a long time that severe obesity can be associated with excessive fatigue. A very obese boy in Charles Dickens's novel *The Pickwick Papers* suffered from what became known as the Pickwickian syndrome, a tendency to fall asleep at the most inappropriate times. Similar symptoms are found in people who suffer from sleep apnea, a condition where a person fails to breathe adequately during sleep and is excessively sleepy during the daytime. We have noted that even moderate daytime tiredness, however caused, can make weight loss difficult. Tiredness leads to reduced physical movement and, of course, a reduced expenditure of calories. More importantly, *when people are tired they often eat when not actually hungry to maintain their energy level and restore concentration.*

When you are tired, if you choose the right food in the right quantity, such as a cookie, a piece of chocolate, or a piece of pie, you will feel an energy boost that lasts for perhaps an hour and a half. If you choose the wrong food or eat too much—say, a large meat sandwich or a pizza—you will feel more tired and may be fighting sleep the rest of the day. Over time, people who are chronically tired tend to discover which foods give them the best "lift." We are beginning to understand the physiological mechanisms that underlie the effects of eating different foods. We know that food intake usually results in an increased metabolic rate (the increase is known as the metabolic effect of feeding). Metabolic rate rises perhaps 10 percent, and this is sufficient to restore alertness. If a food is too high in fat content, however, several chemical messengers from the intestine tell the brain to slow the body in preparation for sleep. This is one reason why a high-fat meal may make us feel sleepy.

The relationship between fatigue and difficulty in losing weight is of very real importance and has to be taken into account in making weight-loss recommendations. Before I ever give a client a word of advice about weight loss, I routinely ask about sleep problems and daytime tiredness. If a client reports trouble falling asleep or staying asleep, or wakes feeling unrefreshed, feels tired by lunchtime, eats to maintain an energy level, or needs to nap during the day, we recommend a consultation with a sleep specialist to rule out sleep pathologies such as sleep apnea, nocturnal myoclonus (restless legs syndrome), and other sleep problems.

3. Fibromyalgia Syndrome (FMS)

Fibromyalgia syndrome (or FMS) is a relatively recently identified condition that causes constant fatigue, poor sleep, chronic pain that worsens over the years, and changes in mood. This constellation of physical problems is said to affect two percent of the population. Eighty percent of those so affected are women.

There are no clearly identifiable physical causes for FMS. Commonly, sufferers have seen many specialists over a number of years for assessment of abdominal or stomach pains, pain around joints and in muscles, gynecological difficulties such as severe period pain, headaches, and/or depression. Because standard tests show no obvious physical cause for the symptoms, many patients are simply labeled as malingerers or depressed.

Fibromyalgia sufferers are prime candidates for obesity, because food is often used to help relieve the symptoms of pain, fatigue, and depression. A sleep study (a sleep lab evaluation in which the patient sleeps overnight in the clinic while wired to equipment measuring respiratory movements, blood-oxygen levels, and brain waves) can be used to screen for this disease, since the polysomnogram (the tracing of brain-wave patterns during sleep) often shows specific changes in people with FMS. Treatment approaches emphasize the importance of gentle but aerobic exercise and muscle stretching. Help with sleep problems is very important. There is no cure for FMS, but a specialist in the management of this syndrome can do a patient a lot of good and there are some medications that can help with the chronic pain, and poor sleep.

4. Mood Disorders

Research shows that the incidence of psychiatric problems such as depression is higher among people with weight problems, but this association is often wrongly interpreted as indicating that weight loss will cure the mood state. *Treating the mood state is a prerequisite for weight loss*, but weight loss, if it can be temporarily accomplished, rarely gives long-term relief of the mood problem. Mood disorders associated with obesity, such as depression and anxiety, are medical problems as well as psychological ones. We now know that mood states are linked to changes in the balance of brain neurotransmitters and should be regarded as chemical problems requiring appropriate treatment rather than "character flaws." It is virtually impossible for people to moderate their food intake if they are in the midst of even a mild depression, so it is very important to treat mood disorders concurrently with any weight-loss program. I strongly discourage anyone from believing that overweight is the cause of mood problems and that mood disorders will disappear with weight loss. It is true that a large number of people get an initial "lift" from losing weight, but the effect is temporary.

Even with mild depression, mood problems such as anxiety, sadness, and hopelessness can lead to loss of control over food intake. Many people regard eating for "emotional reasons" as a sign of weakness or poor motivation. Clients are often relieved to learn that their overeating is at least partly caused by anxiety and/or depression. Sometimes the knowledge that treatments other than dieting can be used to help them improves their ability to comply with dietary and lifestyle advice. One in every ten men and one in seven women will suffer a full-scale depression in their lifetime. One-third of all seriously depressed patients have episodes lasting longer than two years, and 70 percent of patients don't spontaneously recover from depression within two years. Depression has a cost in socio-economic terms that is at least as great as the cost of hypertension, heart disease, and diabetes. Even after treatment, there is an appreciable relapse rate, with 52 percent of sufferers relapsing within three years of finishing treatment with medication. After recovery there is still evidence of impairment in relationships with friends and family if the depression went unrecognized or was not treated effectively. Many people who do not meet the criteria for a major depression have a lesser degree of sadness that is often marked by anxiety and irritability. This state is known medically as dysthymia. If these feelings have been present for years, as is common where mood change has evolved slowly, people may not be able to see themselves as depressed or irritable. In evaluating clients, I ask a number of questions about mood issues and, to a lesser extent, use psychological tests to measure the degree of mood disorder. When I feel that a person's mood is a complicating factor, I have to treat the mood problem or refer the client to a psychiatrist if the depression is unusually severe or proves refractory to standard medication. It has been proven to my satisfaction over and over again that mood problems have to be identified and treated along with weight problems or the patient will not progress.

Though this book is not about treating mood disorders, I think it important for patients to know that all but the mildest long-standing depressions (lasting more than a few months) require pharmacological treatment. Many people shy away from medication in favor of psychotherapy because of an unreasonable fear of being addicted or controlled by the drug. Neither of these worries is the least bit valid where treatment is correctly applied. My experience is that psychotherapy is much more likely to succeed where major mood disorder symptoms (sleep disruption, poor concentration and memory, apathy, inability to take pleasure from life events, and thoughts of despair) are first relieved by the use of an appropriate antidepressant.

There has been a good deal of criticism over the use of medication to facilitate weight loss. I discuss the use of diet pills (anorexiants) in chapter 9. However, it is relevant to note here that pharmacological treatment of even a mild level of depression results in weight loss in a substantial minority of people *independently of any diet plan*. This finding reinforces the suggestion that adequate treatment for mood problems should be an integral part of any weight-loss program.

5. Chronic Pain

Chronic pain is an additional cause of weight gain and makes weight loss very difficult. Pain can be associated with many medical conditions, but in my practice the most common cause of chronic pain is osteoarthritis. This is the aching pain that occurs where a joint has been damaged and the cartilage worn down and ligaments overstrained. This "old-age" type of arthritis is seen in relatively young people whose joints have had to carry a lot of excess weight over the years. It is common to have an overweight forty-five-year-old come to the clinic with arthritis in both knees. Often the arthritic pain seriously limits mobility. Such people understand very well that losing weight will help reduce stress on their joints, but they need treatment for their pain so that they can begin to move more freely and burn calories more efficiently. Unfortunately, many overweight people, and sometimes their doctors, feel that because their condition is "self-caused" they have to accept the pain passively. A belief that their pain is in some way "deserved" deters some overweight people from pushing for the best possible pain management. My advice to such people is to stop seeing their obesity and related illnesses as a "punishment" for "self-indulgence" and to get out there and advocate for the best care. Physical movement is essential to losing weight, not just because it helps burn calories but because it lessens appetite if done before a meal, reduces the likelihood of unessential eating, reduces stress, reduces anxiety and depression, and strengthens the muscles that act as protective structures around joints and prevent further joint damage.

It is pointless for doctors or well-meaning friends and relatives to urge a person with chronic joint pain to exercise until pain relief is arranged. Applying ice to sore joints or tendons, massage, adequate stretching before and after activity, Tylenol, non-steroidal anti-inflammatory drugs (NSAIDs), glucosamine, acupuncture, and even slow-release narcotics such as codeine or oxycodone, can all be used to treat pain aggressively and safely in properly selected patients.

The Case of Sarah

Sarah, age twenty-four, had a complicated history. Her weight gain had started after a serious injury to her lower back in a car accident when she was nineteen. Several of the vertebrae had been broken, and she had constant pain in that area. She also had fibromyalgia syndrome (FMS). In FMS there is reported to be an increase in a neurochemical, substance "p," in the cerebro-spinal fluid, and the area of the brain that processes pain messages has a reduced blood flow. Fatigue is a common symptom, and many FMS sufferers are exhausted all the time. Sarah only had energy to move about between 10:00 a.m. and 2:00 p.m., a time window that is characteristically seen in people with FMS. The rest of the day she could do little, and certainly couldn't work or go to school. Not surprisingly, Sarah was depressed and, when I saw her, perhaps 100 pounds (45 kg) overweight.

As she was on a less-than-optimal dose of an antidepressant prescribed by her GP, that was gradually increased and it seemed to improve both her mood and her energy level. She was in constant pain from her back, but said that she didn't feel it as much anymore because she was used to it. She used Tylenol and Advil on and off but acknowledged that they didn't do much, and other non-steroidal anti-inflammatory drugs (NSAIDs) upset her stomach. I knew that if she was going to lose weight she had to move about more, so managing her pain to improve her mobility was essential even if she said she was "used to it."

In clinics dealing with FMS there is little enthusiasm for trying to treat the pain with drugs; however, in selected cases, I think there is a role for pain medication. The approach currently thought best is to re-educate the brain to perceive pain differently by exercising each part of the body very gently. Aerobic exercise is very important. Ensuring adequate, restful sleep is also a major treatment objective, and some people need medication to assist their sleep pattern. Sleep studies are done to determine if someone is a candidate for supplemental air or other measures, including drugs.

We decided to see if Sarah's food control and overall condition could be improved by treating the back pain she had become inured to. We knew that the back pain was *not* part of the FMS, since there was a real injury to the tissues and bones of the back, while in FMS, the body parts that hurt do not show any signs of injury. I suspected that she was using a fair bit of mental energy just coping with the pain of her back injury and that this mental energy drain was contributing to her need to eat excessively.

Candidates for long-term pain management have to be evaluated carefully. It is now thought to be acceptable to aggressively treat chronic pain not due to terminal illness where the pain is *significant, not responsive to ordinary pain measures such as Tylenol or NSAIDs, and where the person has no history of abusing drugs or alcohol (these are the guidelines approved by the Ontario Medical Association [OMA]).* Sarah fit the bill and was eventually stabilized on slow-release oxycodone. She had a very good response and soon reported that she hadn't realized how much pain she was in until after it was gone. The FMS pain is still present, but not the pain in her back. Lessening this one type of pain improved her sleep and mental outlook and made it possible for her to go for a daily walk. To her surprise, her FMS pain felt less severe, her appetite is significantly reduced, and she has begun to lose weight.

Quite a few obese people have similar problems with chronic pain that is not effectively managed. It is self-evident that people with severe arthritis pain in both knees will likely have less pain if they lose weight, but it is difficult for someone in real, chronic pain to lose weight without effective help for the pain. If the joints cannot be treated or replaced, and pain is constantly getting in the way of weight loss, the pain needs to be treated more aggressively. Experience shows that properly evaluated patients do not get addicted or overuse their pain medication.

6. Binge Eating Disorder

Some people—and I believe their numbers are increasing as we get better at making the diagnosis—are overweight because they episodically lose control over food intake. The binge meal is composed of a number of high-calorie food items eaten in large quantity over a short period of time. Episodic binges are much more common than the other classical eating disorders, anorexia and bulimia. In binge eating disorder, there is no purging or laxative abuse, and no hyper-exercising. Many overweight men are binge eaters who have never realized that they were bingeing or that they had an eating disorder. Such people have to gain control over the impulse to binge before they can lose weight. Medication can be very effective in helping them do so, and two drugs are of proven value. These are Prozac and Zoloft. Several others may be helpful, such as Wellbutrin and Effexor.

Weight Loss as a Treatment for Other Medical Conditions

In the preceding section, I discuss the need to treat various medical conditions in order to *achieve* weight loss. This is the opposite of the usual approach, which is to regard weight loss itself as the therapy for treating the health risks associated with obesity.

I have taken this approach because I don't believe you can scare people into losing weight. I don't normally quote dire health risk statistics to my patients to get them to modify their eating behavior or take more exercise. Emphasizing the health risks of obesity and related illnesses seldom motivates patients to lose weight; it usually just drives them away after a short time.

I here are, however, some statistics related to the health benefits of weight loss that it is helpful for patients to know. The fact that a relatively moderate weight loss can dramatically reduce certain health risks can be encouraging and also enable people to set realistic weight-loss goals. For example, modest weight loss, say 5 to 10 percent of starting weight, is distinctly beneficial in the medical management of both diabetes and high blood pressure (hypertension). Here's how.

1. Diabetes

The majority of patients who develop diabetes in adult life are known as type-2 or adult-onset diabetics, and 80 percent of these are overweight. The diabetic state in the adult obese person is different from that of a person who becomes diabetic abruptly, often at a young age and at a normal weight. Such young, early-onset diabetics require insulin injections to stay alive, while the obese adult diabetic has *too much insulin* in the bloodstream. The obese person's problem is that insulin is not able to work properly on body cells for reasons we don't fully understand. The insulin-dependent, normal-weight diabetic does not make enough insulin to allow body cells to metabolize carbohydrate effectively. This is because insulin-manufacturing beta cells that are resident within the pancreas and which make insulin in response to the body's needs have been attacked by white blood cells of the immune system and destroyed. The trigger for this is not fully understood. Thus, the body's own immune system causes diabetes by wiping out the beta cells in the pancreas.

In most obese people with diabetes, however, the picture is radically different and far more amenable to cure because the pancreas and its beta cells are alive and able to make insulin. With weight loss and dietary change, the obese type-2 diabetic can, in many cases, get back to a normal blood-insulin level and a normal blood sugar. Often, as little as a 10 percent reduction in body weight can reduce or eliminate an abnormal blood sugar by normalizing the action of insulin. The goal with obese diabetics is to achieve "metabolic fitness," that is, normal values for blood pressure, blood sugar, and blood lipids. All too often, however, unrealistic goals are set and the diet causes intolerable stress. Diabetes-linked obesity should be managed no differently from any other overweight problem. That is, identify the causes of poor food control and deal with any medical conditions that are making weight loss difficult. One added note: the incidence of bulimia and of binge eating disorder is higher in insulin-dependent diabetics than in the general population, resulting in the development of obesity in some cases. This can make weight management more challenging.

2. Hypertension

Almost 80 percent of hypertension occurring in normal-weight persons is "idiopathic"—that is, it has developed for reasons we do not understand. In overweight people, however, we know that hypertension can occur for several reasons. The first is that extra weight can cause an elevated insulin level, which in turn causes the kidneys to retain salt and water. An increase in blood volume results, with more fluid present in blood vessels, and this in turn raises the blood pressure. A second cause may be that poorly controlled diabetes causes kidney damage. As the kidney is one of the key organs controlling blood pressure and blood volume, damage to it can lead to elevated blood pressure.

In overweight people with hypertension, blood pressure will often return to normal with moderate weight loss. Therefore, the first step is to lower blood pressure to a safe level, perhaps with medication, and then to plan weight loss to a point that allows the medication to be discontinued. The loss of *just 10 percent of current weight will often bring blood pressure back to normal* where complicating factors such as kidney damage have not occurred. The more modest the weight-loss goal, the more likely the patient is to succeed. Reducing the patient's normal calorie intake by 500 calories per day will often do the trick. A 300 pound (136 kg) man does not need a 1200-calorie diet. A 2400–2600-calorie diet will work fine, and is much more likely to be followed.

At the risk of seeming repetitious, I cannot emphasize too strongly that it is *never* advisable to prescribe a "punitive" diet regime (one very much below the patient's current dietary intake). Most patients can't adhere to them for long enough to achieve their goals. Moreover, I believe these diets can result in a worsening of weight-control problems. I discuss this issue at greater length in the next chapter.

7. Cutting Some Popular Diets Down to Size

There are countless weight-loss diets, but no really effective ones. Diets do have a seductive appeal, however. They often appear to offer a simple, quick way to lose weight—a powerfully attractive idea. In the short term, you may succeed in losing weight on one of these diets. In the longer term, however, there is roughly a 90 percent chance that you will regain the weight—and more—after two years.

Diets fail for several reasons, but one major one is that they focus on symptoms rather than causes. They do not appear to help people adopt a healthier diet or permanently improve their control over appetite and food intake. The best way to make this clear is to describe several well-known dietary approaches, explain what they try to do, and discuss some of the effects they have been known to have on people who follow them.

1. Balanced Low-Calorie (Hypocaloric) Diets

The majority of diets promoted by commercial weight-loss businesses are low-calorie (hypocaloric) and balanced, meaning that the number of calories provided is calculated to be quite significantly less than is necessary to maintain your current weight. An example of such a diet would be one that employs *Canada's Guide to Healthy Eating* as a basis for determining the relative amounts of protein, fat, and carbohydrate, and which provides perhaps 1200 to 1400 calories daily. Such a diet generally gives the consumer an adequate amount of protein, much less fat than they were used to eating (usually less than 30 percent of the total calories), and a fairly high level of carbohydrate with a high proportion of fiber. If you adhere to such a diet, you *are* highly likely to lose weight. However, following such a diet actually teaches you to ignore hunger signals, and the diet seldom takes into account the sort of food preferences you had before dieting became necessary. The premise these diets operate on is that if you are shown how to lose weight, and if you are taught how to ensure the right sort of balance among the four food groups, you will not regain the lost weight when you return to eating at a maintenance level. The problem is that very few people manage to diet and then stabilize at a maintenance food intake. All the studies show that, after following a balanced low-calorie diet, people are *less* able to decipher hunger and fullness signals and less able to regulate their food intake than before they dieted. In my view, then, these diets do a disservice to many people.

In my clinic, we work towards a dietary intake of calories that will maintain the weight the patient can *reasonably be expected to get to*, not the weight he or she should be at according to weight-height tables. For example, if a woman is 5 feet, 4 inches (162 cm) tall and comes in to the clinic with a weight of 250 pounds (113 kg), she will virtually never reach a weight the tables suggest is correct for her (125 pounds [57 kg]), without gastric surgery and maybe not even then. If we set a correct calorie intake for a 125 pound (57 kg) woman, perhaps 1800 calories, I know for certain that she will not be able to adhere to it for long. Even if she did, she would lose her ability to decipher hunger and fullness signals, which in the long term are a necessity for weight control. Unfortunately, diet centers often set diets for these people at 1200–1500 calories. The correct approach is to have a food intake calculated to maintain a body weight of 200 pounds (90 kg), because that may be attainable. Weight-loss clinics should be aware that almost all such patients are slowly gaining weight (5–10 pounds [2–5 kg] a year) when they are first seen and hence would be eating, in this case, perhaps 2800–3000 calories daily. A correct weight-loss diet would contain roughly 2300 calories, assuming some level of daily activity such as thirty minutes of walking.

2. Unbalanced Low-Calorie Diets

These diets are constructed by emphasizing protein, or carbohydrate, or fat. Because they emphasize a particular food group, they tend to be simple and easy to follow. One such diet recommends that certain foods not be eaten with other foods because, it claims, the interaction between these foods will be unfavorable for weight loss. Such claims are not based on scientific fact, and the diets are almost always deficient not only in major nutrients such as protein or calcium but in the minor or micronutrients as well. A diet that is high in fruits and vegetables and that prohibits fat, oils, dairy products, and sugar will be deficient in important nutrients such as iron, essential fats, fat-soluble vitamins, and calcium, to name just a few. Other diets are based on the theory that a lower proportion of carbohydrates (usually less than 30 percent of the calories) and a higher proportion of protein and fat is best. However, seriously restricting carbohydrate may cause ketosis. Ketosis is a metabolic state wherein the body is forced to burn fat and protein as fuels. For your body to make sufficient energy to function, the degree of fat oxidation must rise quite high. There is, however, a set rate at which fat taken from body stores can be oxidized (used up by cells to provide them with energy). If the rate of fat metabolism (oxidation) exceeds the limit the body can accommodate comfortably, liver cells make the fat into chemical molecules known as ketones. These ketones are then used as a fuel by body cells. The problem with ketone-forming diets is that they can deplete the body of essential minerals such as sodium, potassium, magnesium, and so forth. These diets have enjoyed some popularity because the ketone production is thought to reduce the feeling of hunger, but there is no evidence to support this belief. *They are also popular because they cause very rapid weight loss, but this is due to dehydration and that is dangerous.* Such ketogenic diets can be unsafe and are deficient in many elements unless adequate supplements are given. Very few non-specialist doctors and virtually no diet counselors know how to set these diets up with the correct level of supplementation, particularly if a patient has medical problems or is on medication.

These diets can also cause nausea, constipation, low blood pressure, fatigue, menstrual irregularity, headaches, and electrolyte imbalances leading to heartbeat irregularities.

3. Protein-Sparing Modified Fasts (PSMF)

In the early 1970s, there was a vogue for the "Last Chance Diet," a liquid diet composed of a poor-quality, incomplete protein (liquified collagen, which is derived from animal tendons, skins, hooves, etcetera), little carbohydrate, a bit of flavouring and salt, and essentially no fat. It had far too few of the essential minerals (electrolytes) such as sodium, potassium, and magnesium. People lost a lot of weight on this diet, but seventy people died of sudden-onset cardiac failure within several years. Medical science has since learned more about the dangers of these diets and the problems people encounter when they try to return to normal eating after being on them. Further studies have helped us understand how such diets can be safely developed for carefully selected individuals.

I have put people on modified PSMF (a diet of measured amounts of meat, fish, or chicken, very little carbohydrate, and lots of mineral and vitamin supplements) when they were severely overweight and had dangerous medical problems that demanded rapid weight reduction (conditions such as congestive heart failure or severe hypertension). However, these diets should only be recommended for people who are more than twice their ideal weight and who have failed to lose weight on more balanced diets. Even then, we use such a diet only where there is imminent risk of serious medical problems if weight is not lost quickly. Poorly constructed and inadequately supervised versions of these diets are still being offered, unfortunately, despite the fact that we know they can be dangerous. Such diets come in the form of a solid or liquid food diet with few supplements and inadequate screening before and during the diet. Such diets can usually be found accompanied by injections of vitamins such as vitamin B-12, which are claimed to assist the weight-loss process but are useless. I cannot stress enough that legitimate nutrition practitioners almost never use such diets. These diets are deficient in calcium, potassium, sodium, phosphorus, zinc, magnesium, iron, and selenium, not to mention various vitamins and essential fatty acids.

Some commercial liquid diets are available that are low in calories and fat and have adequate protein, vitamins, minerals, and other nutrients. These commercial beverages are government-approved (have the designation "Meal Replacement") and are safe for use over a short period of time, perhaps one to two months, but only where real food is eaten along with these products. In other words, these replacement meals are not to be used as the sole source of nutrition. However, the problem is that the weight lost is almost always regained plus additional weight.

4. Diet Misconceptions

The weight-loss industry offers many examples of myths that have been promoted to truths. Take, for example, the belief that grapefruit will "burn off fat." A diet based on this myth recommends eating mainly grapefruit for ten days or so. A person following this diet will lose substantial amounts of muscle tissue, something not at all desirable. Another myth is that fasting is a good way to lose weight. Fasting contributes nothing to weight loss and can be harmful, particularly for people on medication or the elderly. Muscle mass is lost in addition to excess fat. Weakness, low blood pressure, fainting, and other side effects make this approach unsafe and ineffective. Other blatant frauds are:

a) The Miami Heart Institute Diet

This diet is composed of a special vegetable soup you make and drink daily to lose weight. It has also gone by the name of the Toronto Heart Diet, the TGH Heart Diet, and so forth. The names of hospitals (including several non-existent institutions) are used, without permission or endorsement, to lend the diet a "scientific" air. There is absolutely no usefulness to this diet and, when used for any more than a day or two, it can be dangerous, causing muscle loss, electrolyte imbalance, weakness, and other unpleasant effects.

b) The Vinegar and Honey Diet

The myth persists that somehow acidic compounds such as vinegar cause fat cells to lose their fat content. There is no truth to this or any similar diet claim. The simple truth is that special foods, either alone or in combination with others, cannot force up metabolic rate or cause fat cells to shrink. Neither can they "detoxify" the body and purge away the excess weight.

c) The Chromium Picolinate-Supplemented Diet and Other Assorted Diet Aids (using minerals, heavy metals [such as chromium or selenium], vitamins, or fats [lipotropic factors, essential fatty acids, conjugated linolenic acid, primrose oil, etcetera])

Here it is claimed that the addition of chromium, hydroxycitric acid (from the plant *Garcinia cambozia*), kelp, and so forth, will speed up fat burning. There is no evidence that any of these compounds increases the rate of weight loss or influences whether predominantly fat is lost or other tissue. These are not "extra-fat-burning" diets; they are a scam, pure and simple, and excess doses of heavy metals can be dangerous.

d) Banana Diets, Beer Diets, Wine Diets, etcetera

In all of these, the marketing ploy is that they will affect metabolism and so speed the burning of fat. Needless to say, these claims cannot be supported.

e) Diets That Use Various Herbs and Claim to Reduce Hunger or Speed Up Fat Burning

These diets include herbal supplements such as Garcinia, ma huang, ginseng, aloe vera, ginkgo, biloba, and the like.

Unfortunately, there is no truth to these diet-aid claims. Furthermore, those that use ma huang, caffeine, phenyl-propanolamine, or ephedra are positively dangerous.

Diets That Are Based on Your Body Type

There has been a vogue recently for self-styled weight-loss gurus to determine what sort of diet is likely to work based on your body's inherent shape. They promote the ridiculous notion that your shape tells you something about the types of foods that are right for you in the weight-loss process. For example, they state that there are specific dietary restrictions depending on whether you are an endomorph (sort of a fire-plug shape), a mesomorph (average body shape with rather a lot of muscle), or an ectomorph (lean and tall). Other approaches involve deciding the correct weight-loss approach for women based on the size and shape of their breasts, der-rières, hips, thighs, or blood type. For obvious reasons, I don't want to give the titles of the books describing such diets, but always remember: *there is no law that makes it a requirement for an author to write the facts. There is no law that requires an author of a weight-loss book to make safe suggestions. Authors can write anything they want, make up any stories they please, and sell these books as guides to better health.* These types of books make good reading if you want humor, but please don't assume they are based on a scientific under-standing of weight problems.

Misleading Advertising

In addition to these frauds, there is a good deal of misleading advertising. The example I discuss with patients most often is that "low fat" does not mean "low calorie." In many cases, a manufacturer may state that a product is fat free and enjoy buyer support because of that claim. Though Hershey's Chocolate Syrup, for example, has never had any fat to speak of, it does have 100 calories per two-tablespoon serving. The new, smart marketing name for it is Hershey's Low Fat Chocolate Syrup. Use of terms such as "smart," "low fat," or "thin" in the name of a product or diet aid can suggest to you that they are good for you, but this is not necessarily the case. "Reduced fat" means that a product has lowered levels of fat compared to the original, but four reduced-fat cookies can still contain 240 calories.

To achieve a good balance of nutrients in your diet, I recommend trying to lower dietary fat to 30 percent of total calories. To do so you have to limit, to some extent, foods whose fat content as a percentage of total calories is well over 30 percent. You can do this very simply by reading labels to check the fat content and avoiding or limiting your intake where the amount of fat in a product provides more than 30 percent of the total calories. It helps to know that 0.03 ounces (1 g) of fat has 9 calories in it. Thus, if a chocolate bar has 296 calories and contains 19.4 grams of fat, 174 calories or 59 percent of the total calories are from fat. In contrast, a store-bought pizza slice contains 290 calories, 0.3 ounces (8.6 g) of which are from fat. This means that 77 calories or about 27 percent of the total calories are from fat. As a snack, therefore, the pizza slice is the better choice from a fat-content perspective. (Remember, however, that if you eat more calories than your body burns off, you will gain weight even if the extra calories are "low fat.")

Specific Examples—Two Very Popular Diets

There are many misconceptions about what makes a diet work. It is often believed that "unique" foods used in the diet contribute to its success in some way. Several diet plans would have you believe that certain combinations of food are more likely to result in weight loss than others. Two of the most popular are the "Fit for Life" diet, and the more recently acclaimed "Zone" diet. The first has as its main premise the idea that combining certain foods is wrong and that weight loss happens best when the "right" foods are taken at the "correct" times each day. This, the authors suggest, is because the human intestinal tract is unable to digest certain foods (such as fats) effectively when they are eaten in combination with other foods (such as carbohydrates). If you don't digest the food correctly, you will be hungry and eat more. However, there is absolutely no scientific evidence to support the theory that we don't digest certain foods correctly if they are eaten in combination with other foods. Humans are omnivores, meaning that we are adapted to eating a wide range of foods. This ability to digest, absorb into the bloodstream, and metabolize all sorts of food is one of the reasons we have survived as a species for almost a million years. Our gastrointestinal tracts are designed to break down all kinds of foods even when they are mixed together. Some people will say that not everything can be explained by science, and that if the diet works there must be some merit to it. My answer is that any diet that reduces calorie intake will, if adhered to long enough, cause weight loss. The Fit for Life diet does reduce calorie intake, but it is nutrient-poor and, if followed for a long time without vitamin and mineral supplements, will result in nutrient deficiencies.

The Zone diet suggests, first, that eating a diet high in protein and low in carbohydrate will "target" your weight loss to the elimination of excess body fat. It also suggests that weight loss is enhanced and appetite is better controlled with this diet approach. Both claims are untrue in the long run for the majority of overweight individuals. The diet was first put forward after an observation in the early 1950s that high insulin levels reduce the rate at which fat cells give up their fat (triglyceride) into the bloodstream. One study took two groups of over-weight people and fed both these groups diets with the *same calorie intake* but very *different nutritional composition.* One group was fed a high-carbohydrate diet (mainly grains, pasta, rice, and fruits) and the other was fed a high-protein diet (mainly meats, salad, and low-carbohydrate vegetables). The group eating mainly carbohydrates lost less weight over several weeks than did the group on the protein diet. This early research was incorrectly interpreted as indicating that carbo-hydrates interfered with weight loss and should be limited in a weight-loss plan. The author of the Zone diet has quoted this same research, but here is why the conclusions are wrong.

When you place someone on a diet that is very low in calo-ries and carbohydrate, the body first uses stored glycogen, a form of carbohydrate made in the liver, as a preferred fuel source from which glucose is manufactured. Over the first three to five days or so of such a diet, the body loses a lot of water (glycogen is bound up with water and, as it is converted to glucose, the water is excreted as extra urine). After as little as two days of severely limited carbohydrate intake, fat is burned as a preferential fuel source and the by-products of fat breakdown, known as ketones, are eliminated in the urine. Ketones are negatively charged particles, and they bind with positively charged minerals such as sodium and potassium. With this mineral–ketone complex goes a lot of water that is lost in the urine. The loss of minerals can be serious, and these need to be replaced.

These two mechanisms, loss of water from glycogen metabolism, and loss of water to eliminate mineral–ketone complexes, cause much of the initial weight loss produced by the high protein–low carbohydrate diet. In addition, the low carbohydrate intake causes a lowering of insulin levels and further water loss because the kidney responds this way to the lower insulin levels. This is why a person on a high protein–low carbohydrate diet seems to lose so much more weight than the person on the carbohydrate-containing diet in the first few weeks. Much of the weight lost, however, is the result of the loss of water and salts. In other words, it is due to tissue dehydration. There is, however, an intellectual rationale for using the high protein–low carbohydrate diet in some people. Lowering carbohydrate intake can lower insulin levels, and lowering insulin levels may make fat cells more ready to give up stored fat for use as fuel. Years ago, it was noted that many overweight people have elevated levels of insulin in the bloodstream. The Zone diet takes this observation and combines it with the flawed 1950s research to conclude that a low carbohydrate–high protein diet will force fat to be used up while leaving "trim" muscle tissue alone.

The truth is that diets of equal calorie restriction, provided they contain an adequate amount of protein (80–100 grams protein or about 8–10 oz. of meat/fish/chicken daily), will yield very similar results over the long term. Body composition is not significantly different with the high-protein (Zone) diet than with a diet consisting of a more normal balance of protein and carbohydrate. While it does not result in better weight loss, however, the Zone diet's high-protein content makes it a more expensive diet to follow.

In its favour, I can say that a minority of people find that a higher protein–lower carbohydrate breakfast, lunch, and dinner do give them better appetite control—that is, less hunger later in the day and less carbohydrate craving—and thus make it easier for them to stick to their diet. Such people can use this diet, provided they take a multivitamin supplement, preserve their calcium intake, and eat enough carbohydrate to avoid ketosis (if in doubt, urine tests can be done to detect ketones).

However, unless they deal with the underlying reasons for weight gain, they are just as likely to regain weight lost on this diet as they are with any other diet.

Weight-Loss "Specialists": Who Should You Trust Your Health To?

I think a word is needed about determining whether the person you see to help you with weight loss is genuinely knowledgeable about the subject. In Canada, the designated health disciplines have licencing laws that restrict the use of terms such as Registered Professional Dieticians (RPDt.) to people who have taken required university training and who have done a hospital internship. Only physicians, registered dieticians, chiropractors, psychologists, or naturopathic doctors, can advertise their names along with these titles. If you consult them with regard to weight loss, they are legally required to adhere to certain minimum patient-care standards and will likely cause you no physical harm with weight-loss suggestions. Often they have had no formal weight-loss training other than being self-taught from books, but they will be honest with you about their qualifications if you ask. However, the commercial weight-loss field is full of people who have essentially no training in nutrition and are not licensed under government legislation. "Counselors" in commercial diet centers have had no legitimate training worth mentioning but are often among the small group of clients who have had some success with weight loss in these commercial centers. That does not qualify them to give advice to others. People who designate themselves as "certified nutrition counselor" or use similar terms are not trained at all other than having whatever teaching they got from their "guru," who may have no professional qualifications in the field. Sales staff in vitamin-herbal remedy stores are often asked to give nutrition advice or to recommend products to assist weight loss. Such advice is worthless, so buyer beware!

Your only guarantee of getting safe advice is to seek out a certified professional who is licenced under government regulation. Your best course is to ask what approach they take to weight management and see if it makes sense. Common sense should always be used. Remember the old adage, "If it sounds too good to be true, it likely isn't true." The guidelines in this book should help you to determine if you are going in the right direction.

8. A More Effective Approach: Finding Out What Works for You

Eight years ago, my colleagues and I recruited fifty overweight people for a study. We hoped to identify some common factors among them that would help us design a new, more effective approach to weight loss. The participants had all responded to a newspaper advertisement asking for volunteers who were willing to pay $350 for a day of medical/psychological interviews, psychological tests, dietetic assessment, body composition analysis, and calorimetry (as described in chapter 4), a test that measures how many calories a day a person needs to maintain his or her current weight). We offered this evaluation at a cost because we wanted to attract "expert dieters," people who had already been motivated enough or anxious enough to seek help from a commercial weight-loss center. In short, we wanted to study people who already knew a great deal about weight-loss programs but who still had not resolved their weight problems. We believed that their insights and experiences would be applicable to every overweight person who has lost weight only to regain it and more.

Our volunteers were carefully instructed over the phone how to keep a record of exactly what they ate (and not to try to curb their food intake in order to "look good") for the week before their day-long evaluation. They were also instructed not to eat after 8:00 p.m. or drink (except sips of water) after midnight of the night before their evaluation. They were to fast the day of the evaluation until after body-composition measurement and calorimetry testing were completed.

These people were all very overweight, with an average Body Mass Index (BMI) of 34 (ideal BMI, WHO standard, is 18.5 to 25). Their average age was thirty-eight, and they were generally healthy except for the obesity. All had been to three or more commercial diet centers, but none had dieted actively in the preceding two months. All were at a stable weight, and none were found to have an active eating disorder on standard psychological testing, though several had had bulimia as teenagers.

We found that all fifty of the volunteer subjects had normal metabolic rates—that is, they all burned calories normally in the fasted and resting state—and so we knew their obesity was not due to an inability to burn calories. A substantial minority had sleep problems suggestive of sleep apnea. And all the subjects had psychological scores for depression and anxiety that exceeded those found in patients of normal weight attending a psychiatric outpatient clinic for treatment of depression. It is important to note that none of these people volunteered information about their feelings of depression or anxiety until after a full hour of questioning about life events, family relationships, job problems, and so on. This is a key issue, because it is commonly reported in the medical literature that psychological distress is *not* a cause of obesity though it may be a result. I don't believe that anymore. As we documented our participants' history of the development of obesity problems, I received the firm impression that their distress was chronic and showed up as feelings of anger, powerlessness, and a sense of loss.

Without exception, these participants had long-term stress in their lives and had responded to their feelings of anger, loss, and powerlessness by eating to soothe the negative feelings. It seemed clear that stress had caused their eating problems, and that their eating problems predated their development of obesity. Why, then, do reports of the psychopathology around obesity downplay mood state as a cause of the development of obesity and its continuance?

I think it is because it can take several sessions to establish trust and allow people to talk about issues that affect their emotions. Few weight-loss clinics have staff trained to make such inquiries, and few physicians or dieticians know of these associations. Fewer still have the time to really ask questions about changes in mood and to look at the two different temporal associations between mood problems and appetite-regulation difficulties. Briefly, a majority of patients can agree that events that cause, for example, anger or frustration, can trigger overeating. In other words, they recognize the direct temporal association between the event and poor eating control. A substantial minority of patients do not see this link. Yet, if we get them to chart mood state and eating behavior, not infrequently we see a 24- to 48-hour lag between an event and poor eating control. We think that, during that time, they are mulling over the event subconsciously, and then feeling the upset 24 to 48 hours later.

Clearly there is no shortcut to identifying the root causes of a weight problem. Without such detective work, however, it is difficult to prescribe appropriate treatment.

In our study group, virtually none of the people failed to correctly answer simple questions about diet. There was no one who could not tell me what a good breakfast would be made up of. For example, most people said that a good break-fast would be a bowl of cereal in skim milk, some fruit, and perhaps a piece of toast. Similarly, when asked about a "good lunch" no one had any trouble describing an adequate lunch. An example was often a tuna sandwich, a glass of skim milk, cut-up veggies, and fruit. Similarly with a healthy dinner: all felt that meat or chicken should be eaten sparingly and the fat trimmed off. Pasta was a good choice in limited amounts. Vegetables were a must, either cooked or raw, and fruit was the best choice for dessert, though it was permissible to have cake or pie sometimes. I and my co-workers were impressed by how well many of these volunteers could count calories and by the number who could tell us which foods were high in fat. Most said that they had been dieting on and off for years, and knew very well what they *should* be doing. They just couldn't do it.

Our conclusion? Dietary teaching has little or no effect on long-term success with weight loss, although it can play a lim-ited role where the physician has confirmed that the person truly does not know what elements make up a reasonable diet.

One further very significant finding of our fifty-person study was the evidence that almost half (48 percent) of the people in the study did not record their food intake correctly. According to their seven-day records of their normal diet, nearly half the respondents had an average intake of 1350 calories per day. Calorimetry tests, however, told us that many of these people had to be eating more than 2700 calories a day to maintain their weight. We decided to use the term *under-reporter* to char-acterize this group. (The remaining 52 percent of the study group brought in diet records that were within three percent of what we knew they metabolized daily. We called these people *correct reporters*.) We determined from our psychological tests that the 48 percent who were under-reporters had a distinctly different psychological profile from those who were correct reporters. The under-reporters all were much more "externally focused." They could tell you what everyone in their family expected from them, and what everyone in their office needed from them. They had their "fingers on the pulse of everything" and were expert at finding workable solutions for other people's problems. They also had a very poor idea of when they were hungry and could not easily distinguish between mood states such as anger, sadness, or frustration and physical sensations such as fatigue or hunger. (This inability to identify correctly the emotion being experienced is known as alexathymia.) Lastly, under-reporters consistently failed to correctly judge portion sizes when shown plastic models of foods commonly used. Their inability to judge size meant that they saw large portions as "okay" or average. It is not hard to see how their ability to record dietary intake or to guestimate food intake would be adversely affected.

We concluded that sequential diet records are useless other than for seeing if a person's diet includes a balance of foods from the four food groups. Furthermore, when an overweight person is not losing weight on a supposed intake of 1200 to 1500 calories, the solution is *not* to give the person a diet even lower in calories. Doctors and dieticians who do so are simply misdiagnosing the problem. The patient is failing to lose weight not because of slow metabolism but because of being out of touch with what he or she is doing with food. In other words, such patients will swear to their adherence to the diet, and truly believe they are doing everything correctly, but we know they are not aware of their use of food. We can show the proof of this to a large majority of patients, who will then accept this explanation. They are often relieved to know, finally, why they are failing to lose weight. A few, however, insist they are doing the diet correctly and that there must be some "undiagnosed metabolic" problem that we haven't searched hard enough for. We cannot help such people, although in time they may change their minds and come back prepared to look at the issues.

Why do we spend so much time and money putting people on diets? The vast majority of normal-weight people do not know of or practise a "perfect diet." Yet the most popular method of treating obesity is to focus on diet teaching. Overweight people invariably experience the teaching exercise either as condescending or as a punishment.

Perhaps more importantly, this approach makes the obese person feel stereotyped as someone who lacks willpower and understanding. Virtually all these people understand the elements of a healthy diet, so when the professionals simply repeat things they already know they feel belittled and angry. Very few overweight people fail to understand that lifestyle changes such as getting some exercise are beneficial to weight management. That simple advice, too, they have heard many times. Often, at the end of my first interview with a patient, he or she will say, "I didn't know what to expect when I came. I thought I would be put on some diet or other, so I have actually been overeating this past week. I am really glad no one asked to weigh me. I am relieved that we did something different here, talking about why I can't control my eating better. Will you ever be putting me on a diet?" The answer is *not likely*.

The Treatment of Obesity: A Rational Approach

We have developed a rational plan for doctors, dieticians, and patients to follow in treating obesity. The list that follows draws together a number of ideas that have been discussed in earlier chapters.

1. First, clinically (by simple observation) determine if the level of overweight puts the person at significant risk for developing the medical conditions associated with obesity. It is not usually necessary to weigh the patient to determine this. (If desired, obtain the person's waist measurement, which is a useful indicator of the degree of obesity and correlates well with the risk of developing obesity related illness such as heart disease. A waist circumference above 39 inches (100 cm) for men and 35½ inches (90 cm) for women indicates that a full assessment should be done.)

2. If weight is taken, a BMI of over 27 indicates that a full assessment should be done.

3. Determine whether the person has any of the main conditions that lead to poor control of appetite and lowered mobility: mood disorder, chronic tiredness, chronic pain (including fibromyalgia syndrome), chronic gastrointestinal problems, and binge eating disorder. These issues must be investigated (e.g., a sleep study is essential for an obese woman who has non-restorative sleep and is chronically tired) and treated before there will be much response to dietary measures. Once the main causes of obesity are effectively treated, a significant minority (up to 30 percent) of patients will *spontaneously* begin to lose weight. For example, treating binge eating disorder or depression (with drugs such as Prozac or Zoloft or, in some cases, with cognitive behavioral therapy) promotes weight loss, since clients no longer feel the urge to consume such large volumes of food.

4. Take blood pressure and do lab tests to identify any other medical problems, such as diabetes, high blood cholesterol, and so on. These can and should be treated concurrently with management of the five main causes of weight gain. Management of, for example, high blood sugar, will

improve how the person feels and enhance his or her ability to deal with appetite and activity issues.

5. For the 60 percent of patients who feel better after having their sleep apnea treated, their pain reduced, and so on, but who do not lose weight, it is necessary to determine whether they are under-reporters or correct reporters before proceeding with further suggestions for weight management.

Under-reporters are not lying or trying to deceive the doctor or dietician. They simply can't maintain an accurate focus on the food they consume. Because they are not in touch with what they are doing with food, it is pointless to teach or recommend a diet to them. Cognitive behavioral therapy is needed to put them more in touch with mood and somatic sensations. Unfortunately, few experts in this type of therapy are covered by government health plans.

Correct reporters are much more likely than under-reporters to respond to a structured plan that stresses regular eating (the four-hour rule), stopping a meal before feeling full, and getting thirty minutes of physical activity a day. Correct reporters can distinguish between such sensations as hunger, fatigue, anxiety, and fullness. Therefore they do not need to be put on a 1200-caloric diet. They need some help in making a meal plan that meets their food requirements for their attainable weight. Attainable weight is that weight the person is likely to achieve given his or her age, height, sex, body build, and the duration and severity of the overweight condition. It takes experience to get a feel for what amount of weight a person can be expected to lose. A 20 percent weight loss overall is extremely good, and that is roughly what I have in mind when I begin to discuss amounts of food with a patient.

For example, a 35-year-old woman who is 5 feet, 4 inches (162 cm) tall and has weighed 240 pounds (108 kg) for ten years should weigh 125 pounds (57 kg) or thereabouts according to the tables. However, I would consider she had done a great job by losing and keeping off 40 pounds (18 kg), or about 17 percent of her weight, finishing with a weight of 200 pounds (90 kg). She might not be happy with that evaluation initially, but I have found that, if the goal is properly explained, patients are more comfortable with a realistic assessment of their ability to lose weight. In addition, this woman would have greatly reduced her risk of obesity-linked illness by losing this amount of weight. Commercial weight-loss centers do not make a reasonable assessment of expected weight, and this is one reason they fail their clients; unreasonable expectations cause failure, time and time again.

Up until now I have stressed the reasons why it is important to deal with the emotional and physiological problems that interfere with appetite control and mobility, and the reasons why prescribing a specific calorie-controled diet may be counter-productive. However, while I don't advocate putting people on diets as such, I do recognize that you can't tackle issues of appetite control without discussing the timing and content of meals.

The important point to remember is that any weight-loss plan (plan, *not* diet) must be individualized—tailored to your particular tastes and needs. Therefore, *you* must actively undertake the trial-and-error process of identifying what works best for you. Based on my experience, I offer the following suggestions.

Dietary Approaches That May Improve Appetite Control

I have already discussed why it is essential to eat regular meals, starting with breakfast. In addition, you will find that certain menu plans seem to give you better appetite control than others do. For example, some people find that a breakfast that is higher than average in protein and fat gives them more of a feeling of contentment and fullness than a breakfast that has the same number of calories, but which is made up mainly of carbohydrate. The protein breakfast could consist of two eggs (I recommend the new Omega 3 eggs because their cholesterol content is quite low), a slice of toast with margarine, and some fruit. Another example would be a slice of skim-milk cheese melted on toast or a sandwich of low-fat meat (turkey, roast beef, or chicken) or fish (tuna or salmon) with a glass of milk and a piece of fruit. The carbohydrate version of breakfast would look quite a bit different. A breakfast high in complex carbohydrate could contain bran cereal and milk, fruit, and toast with margarine.

Checklist: Food and Mood Record

This is the form we use in our clinic. It was designed by my colleague, Charmaine Michael, who is our art therapist.

1. To use this record, fill in the times of day meals/snacks are eaten. Note whether you recall being hungry before a meal and whether you felt full afterwards.
2. Indicate whether you did any form of activity that day in the box for "exercise."
3. Mood: At the end of the day, tick off as many of the adjectives you feel accurately describe your average mood that day. Write in any other moods you felt.
4. Control: Indicate whether you felt generally in control of your food intake that day with a "Yes" or "No."

I advise trying one or both of these breakfasts for at least a week while keeping a record of your level of appetite control. The checklist shown here may be used to record food

MONTHLY FOOD/MOOD PROGRESS RECORD

MONTH															
B/FAST															
LUNCH															
DINNER															
SNACKS															
BINGES															
VOMIT															
EXERCISE															
MOOD fine happy motivated relieved sad bored lonely stressed irritable tense angry insecure worried															
CONTROL															

intake, feelings of hunger and fullness, and mood fluctuations. The dietary choice at breakfast that works for you is the one that optimizes food control and leaves you feeling level in mood. The majority of people do best on the balanced breakfast, which is mainly carbohydrate; however, the high-protein (and hence higher-fat) diet can be very helpful in selected cases.

A comment is in order here about *Canada's Guide to Healthy Eating*. No single food group contains all the nutrients necessary for good health, and we do make sure that our

patients recognize the need to eat a mixture of foods from all the food groups. However, I do not agree with the guide's recommended balance of foods. My experience is that eating a diet high in complex carbohydrates, very low in fat, and moderate in protein may leave people feeling hungry and contribute to overeating and weight gain.

My advice is to experiment with varying amounts of fat, protein, and carbohydrates to achieve a mixture that yields the greatest feeling of fullness while achieving a fat content of roughly 30 percent of your total calories.

Creating a Diet Plan That Works

a) Breakfast Is a Priority: The Start of the Four-Hour Cycle of Eating

Turning now to the first step in creating this diet plan, I like to have patients start by making breakfast a priority. If you find that having breakfast upsets your stomach, a snack may be the solution, so that you eat at 7:00 a.m. and again at 11:00 a.m. Eating has to be planned so that *random grazing* does not happen. Eating should happen often enough that *no more than four hours* elapses between a meal and either a snack or another meal. The purpose of this *four-hour rule* is to keep blood-nutrient levels from fluctuating widely during the day. When blood-nutrient levels fall below a set point, hormones are released into the bloodstream to raise the levels. The effect is to make you especially preoccupied with food later in the afternoon and less able to sense fullness even after a normal-sized evening meal.

REMEMBER: **The largest problem with food-use control is not overconsumption at meals, though that can be an issue. Usually, the overweight person indulges in frequent unplanned snacking during the afternoon and evening.**

One of the fears that patients talk about often is that, if they start eating breakfast, they will be more hungry than usual all day, and will overeat. The truth is that eating regularly, beginning with breakfast, simply makes you more aware of hunger, it does not make you hungrier. By eating breakfast you will also find that you are more aware of fullness early on in the meal, and this enables you to choose to stop eating sooner. Within three weeks of regularizing meals and snacks, less food is eaten than before, certainly less than was eaten when most of the food was taken later in the day.

If you have breakfast at 6:00 or 7:00 a.m., you will need a snack by about 10:00 or 11:00 a.m. to keep you within the four-hour rule. Some fruit or a glass of milk will do. A piece of toast is fine, and so is 2% yogurt. You may find it hard to get used to the idea of eating a snack at 11:00 when you will be eating lunch at 12:00 or 12:30. However, once you try this out, you will find that your lunch control is better and you aren't as hungry at 4:00 p.m.

b) Lunch

I find that starting a meal with soup or salad helps in appetite control. Most people enjoy either of these starters and they are low in calories. Main courses for lunch can vary widely, from a simple sandwich to a hot meal. The key for most people who are just starting the weight-loss process is to choose foods you like. It is unhelpful to alter a menu radically to exclude foods that are old favorites or standbys, such as a tuna sandwich, spaghetti, pizza, or a hamburger, just because these are not traditional low-fat diet foods. Certain of your preferred foods may have important associations for you (comfort, lower perceived stress), and these associations can be useful for appetite control. For example, a familiar food may send subtle signals about fullness and satisfaction. Once you have established that a certain quantity of a particular food usually leaves you feeling adequately fed, you can use that information if, the next time you eat that food, you find you want seconds. *Knowing your usual response to a common food may help you control your intake if you pay attention to these signals.* For this reason, I don't agree with the received wisdom that old food habits should be got rid of altogether. Some caution is called for, of course, but most overweight people know that one or two slices of pizza should be enough. Common sense will tell you to have more salad rather than more pizza.

c) Afternoon Snack

It is important to have an afternoon snack planned, particularly if you will be arriving home from work at snack time. For most of us, the snack will be needed at about 4:30 p.m.—that is, four hours after the end of lunch. If you leave work at 5:00, the snack will be eaten before you leave for home. The snack prevents you from being so hungry while you are making dinner that you feel the urge to nibble. If the snack is for someone coming home from school, it should be made the night before, or at least in the morning before going to school, and left in the fridge. The ready-to-eat snack prevents the sort of foraging that goes on when most teenagers come in the door from school. This is a time when overeating can easily occur. A planned and prepared snack could be a glass of milk and a couple of oatmeal cookies, or four crackers with cheese, or a 6 ounces (175 g) container of 2% yogurt with the fruit in the bottom.

It is during the afternoon that many people eat to sustain their energy level. It is important to have a snack rather than a mini-meal at 4:00 p.m. To avoid excessive food intake, when you are tired and having that mid-afternoon slump, walk after the snack. Physical movement should accompany efforts to regain energy at this time.

If you are tired when you come home, try to have a shower or bath after your snack. If possible, read a book, close your eyes for a mini-nap, or listen to some music. *But don't eat more to regain energy.* If this doesn't work, discuss the problem with your doctor. You may be hyper-somnolent or excessively tired because of a sleep disorder or other medical problem. It is worth spending quite a bit of time finding out what will work if you find you need excessive amounts of food in the afternoon to keep your energy level up. Low blood sugar (hypoglycaemia) is very rarely the cause of this tiredness, though it is often blamed because a good hit of sugar re-establishes energy. As a rule of thumb, if you could fall asleep during the daytime within five minutes of being in a comfortable chair, you are too sleepy and it is likely not normal. In an obese person *especially*, it requires an evaluation.

d) Dinner

As with lunch, starting dinner with soup or salad is a good idea. I advocate eating from all food groups at dinner, so that means a good helping of vegetables. It is advisable to set some limits for starch intake, as most people are a bit too free with their servings of pasta, rice, or potatoes. A reasonable amount of rice or pasta would be 5 ounces (150 g or two-thirds of a cup) if it is used as a side dish and 10 ounces (300 g or one and one third cups) if it is used as the main course (a rice pilaff, for example). Meat, chicken, or fish should be limited to the amount that will fit on the palm of your hand, roughly 4 ounces (115 g). Salad, veggies, fruit, and liquids make up the balance of the meal once the starches have been put on the plate. (Remember that the amounts of food shown here are only to indicate relative proportions of food items so that the dinner plate is balanced in nutritional terms. The food quantities need to be increased proportionately for people who weigh a lot more than they should.) A dietician or physician can calculate the correct calorie intake to achieve slow weight loss using the following equations:

Table 8.1:
Calories Needed to Maintain Current Weight

Males:

Age	Basal metabolic rate (BMR)	× 1.50 = approximate calories needed for weight maintenance
18–30	15.3Wt* + 879	
30–60	11.6Wt + 879	× 1.50 = maintenance calories
60+	13.5Wt + 487	

Females:

Age   Basal metabolic rate (BMR)

18–30   14.7Wt + 496
30–60   8.7Wt + 829   } x 1.50 = maintenance calories
60+   10.5Wt + 596

---

*Wt = current weight in kilograms

SOURCE: World Health Organization, *Energy and Protein Requirements*: Report of a Joint FAO/WHO/UNU Expert Consultation Report, Series No. 724 (Geneva: WHO, 1985), p. 71.

Example: A female age thirty who weighs 220 pounds (98 kg) and is obese. Her calorie needs to maintain current weight are 14.7 x 100 kg = 1470 + 496 = 1966 calories x 1.50 = 2949, assuming she is engaged in light activity during the day (i.e., 75 percent of waking time spent sitting or standing and 25 percent spent standing and walking). If a subject sits more than this I use the factor of 1.35 instead of 1.50, to multiply BMR.

For weight loss, we recommend a diet roughly 500 to 700 calories less than the maintenance requirement—in this case, a diet of about 2200 to 2400 calories. Activity level should be raised if possible to burn more energy.

As I mentioned earlier in this chapter, this structured plan based on the "four-hour rule" can work quite well for people who are aware of what they are doing with food. The real key to weight control, however, is being able to stop eating before you are even close to being full. This requires you to recognize when you are *close* to being full. This can be taught, and it helps to internalize the mechanism of weight control more effectively than diets, as such, can do.

In essence, what a person needs to do during the meal is to eat slowly enough to recognize the point at which hunger is disappearing, and fullness is not yet apparent. For example, a person may have eaten a starter salad and begun the main course, perhaps a chicken breast with mashed potato and two cooked veggies. As he works his way through the food items, he ought to become aware that:

- the taste of the food is lessening in its appeal and in its appetite-stimulating effect;
- the sense of urgency to eat is decreasing;
- the sense of hunger is lessening progressively until it is almost gone.

All of these feelings usually occur before any fullness is felt. I tell patients to experiment with stopping the meal when they note the above sensory changes or the appearance of a hint of fullness. This internal awareness takes weeks to work on, but I really believe it is the only long term means of controlling weight.

Once the feeling of faint fullness appears, stop eating and leave the table. If you remain, you are likely to nibble. After fifteen to twenty minutes of reading, doing housework, watching TV, etcetera, check to see if you still feel hungry. More likely, you will feel that fullness has developed to a point where you are satisfied. Satisfied does not mean "fully full"; it means comfortable enough to work or play without noticeable hunger for three or four hours. If you can achieve this amount of control over food, you will lose weight rather easily.

Where the awareness of these signals is more difficult to achieve, assistance from medication may have to be sought. The use of medication in weight control is discussed in the next chapter.

9. Using Drugs in Weight Management

A number of the causes of obesity appear to affect the appetite center, causing an increased perception of hunger, cravings for food, or perhaps a decreased ability to sense fullness. It has therefore made sense to researchers to try to lower people's food intake by modifying their feelings of hunger and of fullness. Several approaches have been tried, usually using drugs that duplicate the effects of such neurotransmitters as noradrenaline, dopamine, or serotonin on the area of the brain that regulates appetite. These neurotransmitter substances can have a variety of effects. Some help reduce the amount of time spent eating, and some produce a reduced feeling of hunger. They can alter food cravings and produce feelings of fullness.

"Thermogenic" drugs have also been investigated. These cause an increase in the rate at which calories are burned up, mainly by increasing the production of heat. Thus, food calories are burned off as heat instead of deposited as fat. Still other drugs have been created that block the ability of the intestine to absorb dietary fat in several ways.

Such drugs have been found to work for some people, some of the time, but their unpredictability is discouraging. It was suggested in 1992 by Michael Weintraub (*Clinical Pharmacology and Therapeutics* 51:5 [May 1992]: 581–646) that such agents have to be safe for use over the long term, as there is no usefulness to giving them for a week or two. Weintraub argued that safe diet pills should be used in the same ways as drugs to treat high blood pressure. In other words, the prevailing habit of prescribing a short course of diet drugs made no sense, since appetite modification has to be a long-term treatment goal. Prior to Weintraub's research, the diet drugs were used for only a few weeks at a time, even though the newer ones, such as fenfluramine and phentermine, were clearly not addictive. Probably because obesity was still viewed as a personality prob lem—a problem of willpower, and hence not a medical issue in the "true" sense—only short-term use was considered. This practice began to change when Weintraub and others tested different agents alone and in combination in order to develop several new approaches to drug therapy.

The Ill-fated Fen–Phen Combination

For about ten years, until recently, there was considerable interest in the use of fenfluramine, pioneered by Weintraub, and then the "fen-phen" combination of drugs. This combination consisted of a drug known as dl-fenfluramine, which stimulated serotonin release and blocked its re-uptake into brain cells, and an agent known as phentermine, which was similar to amphetamine but without its addictive effects. When these two drugs were used together, along with a diet, weight loss was more pronounced than if the drugs were used alone or not used at all.

The average person in Weintraub's studies was treated for over a year and achieved a sustained weight loss of about 15 percent of starting body weight by the twenty-fourth week of the study. There were no serious side effects noted in the studies. One conclusion he reached was that in patients with a Body Mass Index (BMI) of over 30 (or of 27 or more if the person had complications of obesity) these drugs in combination were safe and effective and, in promoting weight loss, decreased the risks the patient faced by remaining seriously overweight.

However, the fen-phen combination produced some mild side effects (such as drowsiness, diarrhea, weakness, or headache) in an appreciable number of patients, making it unlikely that they would use the drugs properly over the long term. A new drug, dexfenfluramine, or d-fenfluramine (Redux™ in Canada and the United States), was made as an improvement over the older dl-fenfluramine. It offered the same weight-loss effects but with a reduced likelihood of side effects. In studies done over a five year period, dexfenfluramine has been effective in assisting weight loss, with just over 30 percent of users reporting weight loss of at least 15 percent of starting body weight. More than 50 percent of users had weight loss of 10 to 15 percent. The placebo group, which got the same exercise program and diet therapy but no active drug, did not do as well. As well as the reduced frequency of the side effects seen with the older dl-fenfluramine, it was also noted that, even where weight loss was minimal, dexfenfluramine lowered users' levels of blood lipids and blood sugars. Though statistically small, these changes were significant because the group that used them was made up of individuals with long-term obesity who had failed on other weight-loss programs. It seemed as though researchers had finally come up with a useful tool against obesity.

Unfortunately, however, a 1997 report in the *New England Journal of Medicine* suggested that almost 30 percent of people using the drug Redux (dexfenfluramine) may have suffered irreparable damage to their heart valves. This has yet to be definitely confirmed, but the drug has been withdrawn from the market worldwide, pending further review. Its partner, phentermine, is still sold and appears not to be connected to heart-valve problems or another possible side effect, pulmonary hypertension (increased blood pressure in vessels leading to the lungs).

Other Agents

There are only four currently prescribable weight loss drugs in Canada—Ionamin or Fastin (phentermine), Tenuate (diethylpropion), Sanorex (Mazindol), and Xenical (orlistat). None have been shown to be more effective than dexfenfluramine. All have the limitation of only promoting weight loss up to a point, generally a loss of 10 to 15 percent of starting weight provided the drug is used indefinitely. It is not thought that these agents lose effectiveness, but clearly some counter-regulatory process occurs in body chemistry/metabolism or in appetite regulation during weight loss, to limit the degree of success achieved. Xenical clearly has added benefit because unlike Ionamin/Fastin and its cousins, it is not absorbed into the bloodstream and hence does not affect the heart or other organs. Its effects and use are described below.

Recently, a new agent, sibutramine, has been approved in the United Kingdom and the United States (Meridia). This drug acts on serotonin and noradrenaline receptor sites in the brain and has resulted in weight loss. Although the jury is still out as to the degree of its effectiveness (so far weight loss is in the range of 15 percent of initial weight), studies show it is helpful, and it may have extra value in the obese and diabetic patient. There is concern that it may elevate the blood pressure in some patients, so care is needed in its use. *Clinical trial studies that I have seen show that it does not improve on the total amount of weight loss beyond what earlier drugs were able to do and it is absorbed into the bloodstream.*

Agents to Hamper the Absorption of Fat

A novel approach to weight management, the blocking of fat absorption, has been achieved with a sophisticated drug, known as Xenical. It was released last year in Europe, and is now available in the United States and Canada. This drug acts by interfering with pancreatic lipase. Pancreatic lipase is an enzyme that is produced by the pancreas and which acts in the small intestine to break dietary fat down into digestible and absorbable free fatty acids. When lipase is partially "disabled" by the drug, roughly 30 percent of the fat in food passes through the intestine and is lost in the stool. Thus, the calories contained in that dietary fat (200 to 300 on average) are not absorbed into the bloodstream. One very significant advantage of Xenical over other weight-loss drugs, is that it is not absorbed into the body, and hence should not have any harmful side effects. Mild side effects can occur if a meal too high in fat is eaten. These include loose stool, cramps, and bloating. The awareness that not complying with dietary suggestions can cause these effects seems to have the beneficial effect of conditioning a person against the use of high-fat foods. In fact, a number of my patients have remarked that knowing that they could have some side effects has helped them stick to the 1800-calorie fat reduced diet recommended by the manufacturer. In general Xenical has no significant side effects if the diet is lower in fat (less than 30 percent of the calories from fat). Xenical also seems to help in the treatment of adult-onset (obesity-related) diabetes. Xenical promoted weight loss in diabetics and in addition, reduced the need for oral diabetic medications that are used in such cases to lower blood sugar. On average, in studies conducted by the manufacturer, weight loss with Xenical is about 20 kg. I have seen more weight loss than that in patients who have had obesity-causing medical conditions treated successfully before starting Xenical. Finally, Xenical is the only drug now available that is recommended for the prevention of weight regain if taken over the long term.

A second non-prescription fat-blocker agent should be mentioned, not because it works, but because so many patients have heard of it. A complex carbohydrate (fiber) derived from the shells of shrimp, it has been popular for a couple of years. This substance, chemically known as n-acetyl glucosamine, goes by various names, such as chitosan. The molecules of this substance develop a positive electrical charge on their surface when exposed to stomach acid in a test tube. When consumed along with a meal, this agent is supposed to form a positively charged gelatinous mass that can attract negatively charged molecules such as free fatty acids to its surface. Some of these fats are said to be absorbed into the chitosan molecule, eliminated in the stool, and not absorbed into the body. There are claims that "hundreds" of calories a day of fat can be prevented from entering the body in this way. These claims are false, though perhaps some fat calories are not absorbed. As one would expect, the truth is that this fiber probably has the ability to lower blood-lipid levels, as any high-fiber diet can, although U.S. studies on this aspect are still pending. As there are no data to support its effectiveness, I don't recommend it.

There have been some concerns that any substance that causes maldigestion of fat, as in the case of Xenical, may lower absorption of important fat-soluble vitamins and certain carotenoids that may fight cancer. Extensive tests on Xenical in over 7000 subjects have not shown this to be true. However, "fat-disabling" methods do not cause weight loss if the diet is high in non-fat calories (i.e., calories from starches), as these calories are not blocked from the body by Xenical. Any diet aid must also be combined with exercise and lifestyle changes to be really effective.

Hydroxy Citric Acid (HCA)

There have been endless infomercials about the benefits of this compound, which is derived from the plant *Garcinia cambozia*. In the test tube, HCA was found to interfere with an important step in the conversion of carbohydrate into fat. It is suggested by manufacturers and sales agents, therefore, that HCA may also interfere with the metabolism of carbohydrate into fat in humans, but there are no studies to show that taking HCA significantly affects body fatness or weight loss in general.

Summary

Medication can never provide a "magic" solution to weight problems. To facilitate weight loss effectively, medication must be combined with a better diet, lifestyle change, and exercise. And not too much should be expected from it. Studies have shown that, on average, it can help you lose up to 10 to 15 percent of your starting body weight. Very few people lose the large amounts of weight so often advertised in the media. In selected cases, however, medication can help produce sufficient weight loss to reduce some of the more serious health risks that result from prolonged obesity.

10. Childhood Obesity: Causes, How to Detect It, and What to Do About It

A six-year-old was referred to me by a physician for management of obesity. The doctor had already advised the parents to reduce treats and limit high-fat foods. The advice had not worked, and the parents and doctor were frustrated. With most such cases, and especially if the child is very young, the first visit is always the same. The child is either unaware that there is a problem or feels he or she is being punished. These kids all look guilty or bored or angry. The parents are frequently overweight themselves.

In taking a history, I ask about developmental issues in the early childhood years, inquire about any serious illnesses, and usually determine that the child is obese but otherwise healthy. I then pursue a few areas of inquiry that are often missed.

1. Were the parents themselves overweight as children? If so, did they remain overweight throughout their childhood and adolescence and on into adulthood? Where this is the case, there is almost certainly an above-average genetic

basis for the child's obesity (likely 50 percent of the tendency to become obese results from genetic inheritance).

2. What is the quality of the relationship between the parents? Children are very attuned to the relationship between their parents, and problems in this area will cause anxiety. In addition, children may blame themselves when parents are in conflict or are separated or divorced, especially (but not only) where the child is quite young (less than seven or eight). Finally, the child may be angry at the parents for not getting along.

   The role played by anxiety, depression, and anger in overeating is the factor most commonly missed in determining why diet advice does not work. Children have as much to be anxious about as adults do, if not more so, and they lack many of the opportunities for dissipating anxiety that are available to adults. Children cannot go out for a drive, arrange to go for coffee with a friend, go on vacation, and so on. They can, however, overeat, ignore parental rules about bedtime, and, as they get older, use drugs and alcohol or get into trouble with the law.

3. Do the parents set a bad example? I am always surprised when parents do not understand that children watch how their parents eat, drink, and so on, and then copy them. Well over half of the obese kids I see have parents who do not eat breakfast, do not exercise on a daily basis, do not eat enough fruits and vegetables, do not get enough sleep, and do not play with their children. I feel particularly strongly that overweight parents should not bring their children in for treatment of obesity unless they are prepared to go along with the same advice I give them for their children.

4. Are other caregivers undermining the parents' efforts? One of the realities of our society is that many children are cared for

by grandparents, nannies, or daycare staff. It is important to know if the rules for eating set down by a parent are being followed by other individuals, particularly by people (such as grandparents) who live with the child. It is quite common for a mother to be trying to modify a child's diet while a grandmother is continuing to feed the child inappropriately.

It is also important to determine if the child is being teased or bullied at daycare or school by other kids. Quite often children who are the butt of cruel remarks from other children will deny that it is happening when the doctor asks. The child is embarrassed that he or she is treated this way by peers and is reluctant to mention it. Parents can talk to schoolteachers and other caregivers to determine whether their child is being bullied. Children need help to deal effectively with bullying. They should get specific instructions about what to do and say when they are bullied or made the butt of jokes.

5. Are rules, including food rules, consistently applied? Here are two examples of parental inconsistency that make it hard for a child to lose weight: (a) When a parent says that certain foods, such as chips or chocolate, are treat foods and must be used in moderation, but changes the rule for no apparent reason; (b) When parents tell their children to eat breakfast, but do not eat breakfast themselves.

Inconsistent parenting is something all of us parents have to struggle against. I have two young boys, and it is hard to remember that being consistent but not a slave to rules requires a very good sense of balance. The books say that kids learn best and feel most secure when a parent is firm, fair, consistent, and loving. This applies to food, too. My kids know that they are allowed treats at birthday parties and so on, but that at home treats such as chocolate are fine a couple of times a week when we have these as a family treat and after a meal. Treats eaten as part of a main meal are less likely to be misused because children's interest in sweets will be less when they have already eaten a main course.

There is no doubt that obesity in children is a health risk. At the Eighth European Congress on Obesity held in Dublin, Ireland, two years ago, childhood obesity was identified as the greatest health hazard facing the industrialized nations and a serious problem even in the developing countries. We don't yet know exactly how prejudicial to future health childhood obesity will be, but we do know in general that the greater the degree of obesity in children, and the longer it lasts, the less likely it is that the child will ever regain normal weight. Fat children become fat adolescents, and fat adolescents have a very great risk of becoming fat adults. It is likely that if a child gets fat enough, new fat cells will be made. Once created, these stay in the body. We know that fat cells signal the brain to regulate appetite to some degree, and it has been suggested that such cells may signal the brain to increase food intake to keep themselves permanently full of fat. If the theory is correct, these fat cells may "fight" weight-loss efforts by sending chemical messages to the brain to increase food intake. This may be one reason why weight loss is so hard once a person has become overweight to the point of obesity.

When we look at the prognosis for overweight kids, it is interesting to note that only 30 percent of obese female teens will ever achieve a return to normal weight, although 70 percent of obese male teens may do so. However, even if overweight young people do achieve normal weight later in life, statistics show that obesity in the first twenty years of life significantly increases morbidity rates in adults over age fifty. Thus there is something about early obesity that sets us on the path to poorer health after age fifty.

If you want to know whether or not to worry about your child, ask yourself if the child *looks* fat. If so, then he or she is probably overweight. Forget the old notion that "baby fat" will just go away. One way of quantifying the degree of the weight problem is to refer to the growth chart the doctor keeps on your child. By recording the weight and height of a child year by year, it is possible to chart the rate of change of height and weight that happens in growing children. Normally, weight and height rise in proportion to one another. For example, a child who is on the 50th percentile for height should be on the 50th percentile for weight as well. However, when a child is on the 50th percentile for height, but on the 97th percentile for weight, there is a problem. Another way to quantify fatness is to measure with skinfold calipers. A pair of inexpensive calipers can be applied to the fat fold beneath the lower pole of the shoulder blade (subscapular location) or at the fold overlying the triceps (see chapter 3, tables 3.1 and 3.2). Of these two sites, the subscapular site gives the best measurement of body fatness. In general, measuring body fatness is the best scientific way to determine if a child is too fat. If the body fat measurement is in the safe-normal range, but the weight centile is more than the height centile, I ignore the weight measurement because the "excess weight" is simply extra muscle or bone, which is harmless.

For example, a teenage girl could be very athletic and have more muscle than average. Her weight could be 140 pounds (63 kg) and her height 5 feet, 2 inches (157 cm). Ordinarily, these numbers would suggest that she is becoming overweight (with a Body Mass Index [BMI] of 25.8); but if her fat-fold measurement was on the 50th percentile—in the normal range—I would not consider her fat. I would tell her that her weight is relatively high, due to extra muscle, and is healthy. I see dozens of referrals each year of teenagers who are not fat but whose muscle mass puts their weight above what the graphs say is normal. Muscle weight is not "dangerous" to health the way excess fat can be.

A word of caution is needed about "late childhood chubbiness." In the year or so before the onset of puberty, many kids become a bit chubby, and this pre-pubertal weight gain is normal. If the child is no more than 10 to 15 percent above ideal weight, the goal of treatment is not weight loss, but rather to see that appropriate ongoing weight gain is limited according to changes in height. Where a child is obese we aim for weight maintenance. In other words, an appropriate goal for an obese child would be to keep the child's weight stable while he or she grows taller or, in other words, grows into the current weight. Children should not be put on diets in the way adults are. Weight loss, if marked, interferes with growth and physical maturation and works against long-term weight management.

When an obese child—that is, a child who is more than 20 percent above ideal weight—comes for help, there are certain to be both emotional and physical issues that have to be sorted out. In their own way, children have at least as much stress in their lives as adults do. At the same time, they have less ability to combat stress than adults.

Children, the same as adults, need a thorough evaluation to determine the possible medical causes of their weight gain, even though their medical problems are usually far less serious than those of the adults. They may suffer from such complaints as upset stomachs, aches and pains of various sorts, headaches, nausea, sleep problems, and moodiness, and these will need to be addressed before any attempt is made to change their eating patterns.

Causes of Excess Weight in Childhood

1. Stress- or Mood-Related Eating

For many years, it has been generally believed in the field of child psychiatry that children don't have the well-defined psychiatric illnesses that adults do. For example, it is not usual to say that a depressed teen has a major depression. Instead he or she is said to have an "adjustment problem" or adolescent moodiness. Whatever the definition, however, mood problems in teens and even young children seem to have reached epidemic proportions. Our society is very quickly changing, there is a lot of stress, and many of the traditional ways of dealing with stress are disappearing. The classic outlet of athletics is a good example. As school gym programs are cut, few parents can afford either the time or the money to set children up in replacement activity programs. Often a child has very little in the way of activity beyond playing briefly in the playground during recess. Kids spend much of their time sitting in class, or sitting in front of the TV or computer. When events happen that make children angry, unhappy, or anxious, they often don't know how to express or get rid of the feeling. Food is a reliable and generally available remedy for feelings such as anxiety, anger, loneliness, and so on. Parents are often surprised to hear that their children are overeating for the same reasons they overeat themselves.

A discussion of how to handle childhood emotional issues is beyond the scope of this book. Help should be sought from experts in the field. (One excellent, readable, and practical resource is Barbara Coloroso's book *Kids Are Worth It.*) I can, however, comment on the handling of weight-management issues. *With a child who is under stress, depressed, or anxious, focusing on the weight problem is the quickest way to lose that child's interest and cooperation in any weight-loss strategy.* Pre-teens and even young teens often know they feel bad (lonely, anxious, scared, or angry) and might acknowledge feeling stressed, but they are usually unable to pinpoint exactly why. A doctor who starts in immediately talking about diet manipulation and weight loss will appear to be just like all the other adults, including the parents, who don't try to identify the *origin* of the child's troubles with food. Even though excess weight may be perceived as a problem by the teen, *at the subconscious level weight loss ranks quite far down the list of items to be wrestled with*. Research shows this to be the case with adults, and I have no reason to believe children are any different. I therefore apply the same rule to both children and adults: issues related to anxiety, depression, loneliness, social ostracism, and so on must be dealt with before weight loss becomes a realistic goal.

2. Mealtimes That Are Not Planned for Optimal Hunger Management

A fair number of the kids I see are fat because their parents are trying to live with a very difficult work schedule and want to have meals together as a family. Suppose, for example, that one parent—say, the father—works nights and gets home at 2:00 a.m. He leaves for work at 6:00 p.m., but wants to have dinner with the children first. Dinner is made and served by 5:00 p.m. When the children get home from school at 4:00 they are hungry, but are told not to have a snack because it will "spoil" their dinner. By the time they have dinner, they are too hungry to have good appetite regulation. They are finished by 5:30 and by 9:00 p.m. are hungry again and eat what amounts to another dinner. From an appetite-control perspective, it would be better for them to have a snack at 4:00 p.m. when they come home from school, and eat dinner around 6:00 or 6:30. The challenge is to find a way for them also to join their father at supper. One possibility might be for them to eat their salad with their father, and have the rest of their meal at 6:00 or 6:30.

Another type of disruption occurs when parents get home at 7:30 p.m. or later. The children may be fed dinner by a relative or at daycare at 6:00 p.m., and then eat again when their parents are having their own supper. The kids will, in effect, have a second dinner.

3. Excessive Use of Treats and Overfeeding

Kids are exposed to the same ads for junk food that adults are and will eat it just as often, if they can. I often find that the diet records of an overweight child show two or three "treat" foods a day. Examples of treat foods are chocolate bars, a bag of chips, french fries, a slice of pie, a regular soft drink, or some chocolate-chip cookies. In general, treat foods should be eaten only after a meal, as a dessert, when the appetite for food is already reduced. *Three treats a week is the normal limit.*

Overfeeding often occurs when children are encouraged to "clean the plate" or are *rewarded* for eating all their food or punished for not eating various foods. A better way to handle kids' meals is to put healthy food servings in front of them and then to *leave them alone.* Children should not be forced, or even encouraged, to finish everything on the plate if they do not wish to. Many parents believe that if they do not push the child, he or she will not get some important nutrients. In fact, that concern is not valid. Studies of children's dietary intake, averaged over a month, show that when left to determine their own intake the vast majority of children more than meet their nutritional requirements, provided healthy food choices are served to them. A child who does not eat much dinner may be allowed a bowl of cereal later on if he or she requests something to eat. You do not have to make the child a new dinner.

4. Genetics

It is estimated that the tendency to be overweight is 45 to 55 percent genetically determined. What this means is that if one parent has been obese since childhood, the risk that his or her child will be overweight is roughly 40 percent. If both parents were obese from childhood onwards, the risk rises to 80 percent. This is one reason why the World Health Organization recently declared obesity to be a disease, rather than a "condition." That means it is an illness with definable origins and symptoms, associated with other illnesses such as hypertension, indicating a need for medical treatment, and so on. We cannot change genetic inheritance, but we can change diet and activity level to compensate. Parents who are fat and have been so from early childhood have experienced the ridicule and social ostracism obesity has caused them. They are generally very willing to try and set a good dietary example for their children and to increase their own activity levels as a way to teach their kids that activity is a key safeguard against excess weight. I would also suggest, however, that if you feel genetics are against you and you see your child gaining even a bit too much weight, it might be advisable to check with a dietician to be sure you are serving correct portion sizes of starches and proteins. (Example: we suggest a limit on starch servings, such as rice, to 2/3 cup as a side dish, or 1-1/2 cups as a main course [e.g., a bed of rice on which is placed some stir-fry beef and vegetables]. Protein in the form of meat, fish, or chicken is limited to about 4 ounces (115 g) cooked weight. For children under the age of five, these amounts are reduced.)

11. Special Conditions That Affect Weight Control

Weight gain may occur under a variety of special circumstances that make standard approaches to weight management inappropriate. These circumstances include pregnancy, mental or physical disability, and dependence on certain drugs used to treat particular medical conditions.

Pregnancy

Not infrequently, my clients include women who want to lose weight before becoming pregnant, or overweight women who have become pregnant and want to avoid further weight gain during the pregnancy. There is no doubt that obesity can reduce fertility. It also complicates pregnancy by increasing the likelihood of diabetes and high blood pressure. Labour and delivery are also more difficult and risky for both mother and baby when Mom is significantly overweight.

It is helpful to evaluate women early in their pregnancy to see if their diets can be modified to cause some weight loss or to improve an abnormal blood-sugar profile. The fetus draws relatively little in the way of nutrients from the mother before the fifth month of gestation. Hence, a diet set to maintain a weight 20 percent or so less than the current weight may be prescribed. The diet must preserve the intake of proteins, minerals, and essential fats, and is normally supplemented with vitamins. This diet approach does no harm and may often result in some weight loss. By the fifth month of pregnancy, weight gain must occur; a total gain of 16 to 20 pounds (7.25–9 kg) seems reasonable in the obese pregnant woman. This gain comes from the weight of a larger uterus, the growth of the fetus, and added blood volume in the mother. Generally, we cannot do much more than slightly limit weight gain, but even that will help. After delivery, breastfeeding helps facilitate weight loss quite a bit if the diet is calorie reduced, and, of course, is best for both mother and baby.

Sometimes—for example, when the mother is depressed—we cannot easily prevent weight gain. Fortunately, mood changes in pregnancy are usually positive. In fact, because pregnancy is generally antidepressant in its effect on mood, some mildly depressed women will recover a normal mood state by the end of the first trimester. Negative mood changes can occur, however. When a depressed mood is bad enough to affect the mother's health, we advocate the use of medication, since there is evidence that serious depression can complicate the pregnancy. The older tricyclic drugs, such as imipramine, are safe in pregnancy, but can increase appetite. Prozac and Zoloft, two of the newer SSRI class of drugs, are safe in pregnancy. When a woman is suffering a real depression, these drugs can be extremely helpful. Helping Mom get better is also a real plus if there are other children at home. Children, especially quite young children, are themselves under stress with the birth of a sibling. There are few things as potentially harmful to the healthy psychological development of a young child or early teenager as a depressed parent who continues being depressed for years.

To sum up: It is usually advisable to help overweight women limit weight gain during pregnancy. Such women should be evaluated carefully, perhaps with calorimetry, and assisted with weight management, particularly where mood problems are evident. It is very important for pregnant women to exercise, and is quite safe if excessive overheating is avoided and hydration is maintained. Swimming, walking programs, low-impact aerobics, and yoga are excellent.

Mental and Physical Disability

When I was training in the field of medical nutrition, I spent quite a bit of time working with children and teens who had cerebral palsy or other mental/physical challenges. Obesity was a common problem with children who were unable to be physically active or who could not express their wishes well enough to make their feelings understood. The more physically and mentally disabled the child or adult, the more often they were overfed in response to movements or vocalizations that their caregiver felt represented hunger. Their vocalizations were just as likely to have signaled discomfort, boredom, tiredness, or anxiety, but we had no way of telling.

The first group I saw with serious weight problems were children with severe cerebral palsy (CP). They were dependent on caregivers for all aspects of day-to-day support, such as feeding, moving, and so on. We studied these patients to determine whether their metabolic rates were less than would be expected based on their weight and height. In the more severely brain-injured individuals, metabolic rate was reduced to much less than expected for their weight, height, age, and sex.

Assessing metabolic rate is important, because doctors or dieticians sometimes make diet recommendations based on the calories a normal child of similar height and weight would need. For these CP individuals, however, such dietary intakes can result in obesity because of the low metabolic rate. Allowance must be made for the fact that the body composition of CP sufferers is different from that of non-sufferers, with a much reduced muscle mass and an increased fat mass.

Other groups with special nutritional needs are people with spina bifida, people who have had damage to their spinal cords resulting in paralysis, and those with a muscle/nerve disorder that limits movement, such as hereditary muscular dystrophy, myasthenia gravis, post-polio syndrome, and so forth. Their problem is similar to that of people with CP. The loss of nerve connection to muscle results in atrophy (shrinkage) of muscle cells. Because muscle is very metabolically active tissue, as muscle mass is lost, metabolic expenditure (the ability to burn calories) falls. Because of their condition, however, these people cannot burn energy by being physically active. In the months after a diagnosis of one of these conditions, it is advisable for the patient to see a nutritionist who can develop a diet that meets protein, mineral, and vitamin needs without being too high in calories.

Avoiding obesity is important with all these disorders, since excess weight causes marked impairment in movement and breathing. The skeletal system may be damaged more quickly where a child with CP is allowed to get very obese.

Medical Use of Steroids

Sometimes people are given steroids such as cortisone or prednisone because they have severe asthma or an auto-immune disease (where the immune system produces antibodies against substances naturally present in the body) affecting one or more organs. In asthma, the tissues lining the airways react, for example, to environmental irritants such as smoke, or perhaps to a viral infection such as the common cold. As these tissues become inflamed they swell, and bronchial smooth muscle constricts around the airways. The diameter of the airways shrinks and breathing becomes harder. Inhaled steroids are used to reverse this process. Occasionally, when the asthma is so severe as to be potentially life-threatening, large doses of steroids such as prednisone are also given, either orally or intravenously, to reverse the inflammatory response in lung tissues. These steroids are not the "muscle builders" people automatically think of when they hear the word "steroid." They are products derived from the adrenal gland, and are normally found in small quantities in our bodies. When corticosteroids such as prednisone are given, they work wonders in dealing with asthma and will usually end the emergency situation and allow a person to leave hospital. However, they have major effects on many body tissues if taken in a high dose for more than a few days. Under the influence of corticosteroid, fat is deposited centrally around the face and abdomen and is lost on arms and legs. The overall effect is a loss of muscle mass and an increase in fat tissue. High doses of prednisone may also dramatically increase appetite, so weight gain, mainly deposited around the central areas of the body, is inevitable. This weight is lost when and if the steroid dose can be reduced.

Prednisone and other steroids are invaluable and should not be feared if prescribed. These drugs are rarely overused or overprescribed by doctors. Where steroids have to be used orally over the long term, weight-maintenance measures should be instituted early, though they may not always be effective because of the sometimes pronounced effect of steroids on appetite. It is also important to maintain bone mass when steroids are used over the long term, and there are drugs that can help with this.

Use of Antidepressants, Mood Stabilizers, and Antihypertensives

Other drugs that may cause weight gain include the tricyclic antidepressants (other than desipramine), the monoamine oxidase inhibitor (MAOI) class of antidepressants, beta blockers (drugs sometimes used in treating hypertension), certain antihistamines, mood stabilizers such as Epival and Tegretol, which are also anti-epileptic drugs, and the mood stabilizer lithium. There are also reports of weight gain with certain SSRI antidepressant drugs such as Prozac, though by far the more common effect is weight reduction.

People who are worried about an increase in appetite or weight while on a drug should discuss their concerns with their physician.

12. When Medical Means Fail: What Other Measures Can —and Can't—Achieve

A variety of non-medical weight-loss approaches have received publicity over the years. As with many "miracle" cures, these are seldom the panacea they may appear to be. Anyone contemplating such measures should be fully informed about their pros and cons. Here are a few guidelines.

Gastric Surgery

In 1954 Drs. Kremen and Linner pioneered stomach surgery to help severely obese people lose weight. This form of treatment alters the gastrointestinal tract so that food cannot be eaten in large quantities and/or bypasses the parts of the bowel where digestion and absorption normally take place. The first surgical efforts involved shortening the length of the small intestine available for the digestion and absorption of food. In this early surgery, the stomach was opened and attached to the last part of the small bowel, known as the ileum. Food would enter the stomach in whatever quantity the person chose to eat, but would then empty undigested into the end of the small bowel, bypassing the parts of the upper small bowel known as the duodenum and jejunum. The overall result was that food was poorly broken down and not absorbed well. Malabsorption of carbohydrate, fat, protein, and many minerals and vitamins often led to serious problems such as malnutrition, liver disease, gallstone formation, chronic diarrhea, and osteoporosis. More recently developed techniques are safer. There are now two main types of stomach surgery performed.

1. Gastric Restriction Surgery

In this approach, the surgeon uses staples to make a small pouch at the top of the stomach where the esophagus enters it (figure 12.1). The volume of the pouch is restricted to about one ounce, and the far end of the pouch is narrowed so that food leaving it passes very slowly into the remainder of the stomach. As you might expect, with such a small capacity for liquid or solid food, the person feels very full quite soon after eating or drinking a tiny amount. In time, the pouch stretches until it will hold perhaps 3 ounces (85 g) of food or liquid, but the far end opening into the remainder of the stomach stays narrow. With this technique, or a modification of it using adjustable bands to alter the pouch volume, patients can lose perhaps 35 to 50 percent of their excess weight in the two years following surgery. Some weight is then usually gained back, but it is rare for all the lost weight to be regained.

2. Gastric By-pass Surgery

This surgery involves making a small pouch at the top end of the stomach as described above, and then attaching the under side of the stomach to a loop of intestine. Thus the volume of

Figure 12.1: Vertical Stapled Gastroplasty

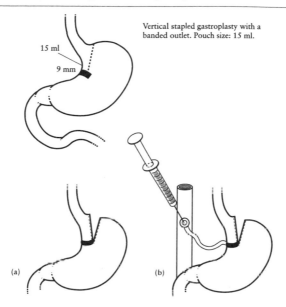

Vertical stapled gastroplasty with a banded outlet. Pouch size: 15 ml.

15 ml

9 mm

(a)

(b)

(a) Gastric banding (b) Adjustable gastric band attached to a subcutaneous port.

SOURCE: G.J. Kral, "Surgical Treatment of Obesity," in P.G. Kopelman and M.J. Stock, eds., *Clinical Obesity* (London: Blackwell Science Ltd., 1988), p. 545.

food entering the stomach is restricted as described above *and* the food that does get into the lower stomach then empties into the distal small bowel, thereby by-passing the duodenum and jejunum where nutrient absorption typically takes place. This surgery therefore both creates a barrier preventing food from getting into the stomach in any but very small amounts (restriction technique or "vertical banded gastroplasty") and produces malabsorption of the food for a "double-whammy" effect. This technique is commonly known as the Roux-en-Y Gastric Bypass. It offers greater weight loss and less chance of regaining weight than the vertical banded gastroplasty process but at increased risk of malabsorption of nutrients causing serious malnutrition. The patient must be monitored for life to prevent nutritional deficiency and will need liquid supplements for life as well. I have seen several patients who had this procedure and none of them feel particularly well or are optimally healthy. We very rarely see this type of gastric surgery done in Canada, though it is popular in the United States.

Who Is a Candidate?

Because all versions of this surgery entail a significant risk, it is important to have potential recipients properly evaluated. Criteria for surgery are:

1. Weight must be at least 100 pounds (45 kg) above the ideal for age, sex, and height for males, and at least 80 pounds (36 kg) for women. (These weights correspond to a BMI of 40 or more.)
2. Full trials of conventional weight-loss approaches, such as diets, medications, counseling, exercise programs, and so on, must have been conducted.
3. There must be evidence that recurrent trials of weight-loss approaches have failed (for example, the regaining of any weight lost).
4. There must be no evidence of untreated endocrine or psychiatric conditions that could be considered causes of obesity. It is especially important for binge eating disorder to be absent or to have been successfully treated before this surgery is considered.
5. There must be no evidence of major illnesses, such as significant and advanced vascular/heart disease, kidney disease, respiratory diseases, or active peptic ulcer disease.

   I also require a thorough psychiatric assessment as a necessary precondition. Having surgery that will dramatically affect how you lead your life is a big step that requires very careful consideration. In fourteen years, I have recommended this surgery to only twelve patients, and two have regained all of the 140-plus pounds (65+ kg) they originally lost.

Risks

There are surgical risks, a variety of possible complications, and also psychological risks.

1. SURGICAL RISKS

Every surgical procedure has anesthetic risk—that is, the risk that death could occur as a result of the anesthetic. Fortunately, this risk is very slight with modern techniques and monitoring facilities. Where appropriate, a very light anesthetic is given along with a spinal epidural block, such as women have in labor, to shut out pain signals. The lighter the anesthetic, the lower the risk of respiratory or cardiac problems. Another risk with surgery is the risk of infection. A hard-to-treat wound infection or peritonitis (abdominal-cavity infection) may occur. Peritonitis almost certainly requires repeat emergency surgery to look for leaks at suture lines, pockets of infection, and so on. Lastly, blood clots can form in the legs after this surgery, and special care must be taken to minimize this risk. A blood clot in a deep leg vein can break off and travel up the vein to the heart and thence into the lungs, causing what is known as a pulmonary embolism. This can be very serious.

2. COMPLICATIONS REQUIRING FOLLOW-UP SURGERY

Ten to 20 percent of patients who have weight-loss operations will need follow-up operations to correct complications. Abdominal hernias are the most common of such complications. Less common are breakdown of the suture line internally and stretched stomach outlets that allow weight to be regained as the feeling of very early fullness disappears. Other risks include adhesions (scar tissue in the abdomen) causing a blockage of the bowel and requiring further surgery, ulcers forming at the suture line between the stomach and the small intestine, and too tight a gastric outlet, causing severe vomiting and dehydration.

3. OTHER COMPLICATIONS

a) Gallstones

More than one-third of obese patients who have gastric surgery develop gallstones. This is because, during rapid weight loss, the rate at which gallstones form increases dramatically. Gallstones may be prevented by taking bile salts (a prescription drug) for six months after the initial surgery.

b) Nutritional Deficiencies

Nearly 30 percent of patients who have weight-loss surgery develop nutritional deficiencies that may result in anemia, osteoporosis, and metabolic bone disease. Low potassium, magnesium, zinc, and many vitamins are other problems. These nutrient deficiencies are much more common with bypass surgery as opposed to the simpler restriction surgery.

(from the International Bariatric Surgery Registry)

In 7415 patients, 10 deaths occurred within forty days of the operation, a mortality rate of 0.1 percent. Complete information for complications and postoperative hospital stay for 4949 patients shows that 91.33 percent of these people had no postoperative complications, while 8.67 percent had complications of some sort. The breakdown by type of complication is as follows:

Risk Statistics for Gastric Surgery

	%
Deep-vein thrombosis	0.2
Gastrointestinal leak	0.1
Subphrenic abscess	0.1
Respiratory complications	3.2
Wound infection	1.1

It should be noted that low numbers such as these are seen only where the surgeon doing the procedure has had many years of experience. The number of surgeons with this level of expertise is quite small, so I would advise a patient to be very sure of the skill of the surgeon before submitting to this operation.

4. PSYCHOLOGICAL RISKS

a) From Lifestyle Changes

Those who have had either form of surgery must alter their eating habits dramatically. They can eat or drink very little at any one time, and therefore need to take nourishment every hour or two. Solid food must be chewed to absolute mush before being swallowed. Chunks of food the size of a peanut can get stuck in the pouch and cause vomiting. In short, this surgery, though effective, will transform your relationship to food and drink. Some people cannot tolerate this. Before such surgery is done, I strongly recommend three things. First, talk with someone who has had the surgery and find out first hand about its impact on his or her life. Some people's experiences are very good; others are just terrible. Second, see a psychiatrist who has helped the surgeon evaluate people's fitness for this type of intervention. Finally, test your own tolerance for the altered eating habits necessary by chewing your food to mush, and eating only 3 ounces (85 g) of food and/or liquid every two hours for a day, to see what it is like. You will experience hunger not felt after the surgery because your stomach has not been partitioned or restricted in volume, but the experience of eating very slowly and chewing the food fully to mush is similar.

b) From Interpersonal Changes

Sometimes when people lose significant amounts of weight, they find that friends and family treat them differently.

For example, new types of demands may be made on them. This new-found attention is often frightening and can provoke serious psychiatric symptoms. Careful inquiry before recommending a patient for surgery should catch this potential problem. Patients who have a phobic weight—that is, a weight they recall having reached briefly that triggered them to feel very fearful and anxious—should have adequate psychotherapy before going through this surgery.

It is not possible to list all of the pros and cons of weight-loss surgery. The best way to explore it is to consult a reputable surgeon with extensive experience in the field. If you have the surgery, make sure that the surgeon puts you in touch with a dietician both before and after the surgery. I am appalled by the terribly poor diets people get themselves on after this surgery because their nutrition isn't monitored after they leave hospital. These diets can be deficient in vitamins and minerals, and in protein as well.

Benefits

This surgery is generally quite effective in assisting weight loss. With vertical banded gastroplasty (restriction surgery), the average patient can expect to lose 50 to 100 pounds (23–45 kg) and sometimes even more. Fifty percent of these patients will maintain the weight loss for five or more years. Without surgery, they would have gained weight at a rate of about 10 pounds (4.5 kg) a year, every year, after crossing the 300-pound (136-kg) weight threshold. Greater weight loss is achieved with the Roux-en-Y Gastric Bypass surgery, and the statistics for weight maintenance are also better, but the patient is at serious risk for malnutrition and has to be nutritionally monitored by a physician and a dietician *for life*.

Liposuction

Liposuction is a method of removing excess fat by vacuuming it out of sites over the abdomen and buttocks or thighs. There are different methods, some now using ultrasonic vibration to liquefy fat cells and make them easier to remove. However, because liposuction also removes a good deal of tissue fluid, including blood, there is a definite limit to the amount of tissue that can be sucked away. The technique cannot be used to lessen leg size below the knee, and, frankly, there is no way this method can safely rid anyone of more than a few *insignificant* pounds of weight.

The procedure has one other very insidious drawback. When fat is removed from one part of the body, a part it normally goes to when weight gain happens, there is no longer any way excess fat can be sent there again because the fat cells are gone. If you gain weight after liposuction, the weight gained will be deposited in a site that is "unusual," and this might be troublesome. Aggressive liposuction can result in serious consequences and should *never* be tried. Stay well away from liposuction weight-loss centers. Liposuction is fine for cosmetic work in selected patients, and that is its proper use.

Hypnosis

Hypnosis has been touted as a cure for overeating. However, although it has been used successfully in helping people to stop smoking or to kick other drug addictions, it is not normally helpful in obesity. It is simply not possible to give people a lasting posthypnotic suggestion telling them not to eat too much. In susceptible people, hypnosis can be used to create a temporary aversion to a specific food, but the effect doesn't last. In my years of practice, I have seen only one patient successfully lose weight after having various food aversions conditioned into him by hypnosis. Hypnotherapy used to assist relaxation and meditation can be useful, however, in people who eat excessively when under stress.

Detoxification Therapies for Weight Loss

There is no way to "wash" fat out of the system, as some of these fad methods claim. *I am particularly against this form of treatment.* There have been no studies to show that fat people (or anyone else for that matter) are "toxic" and needing a "clean out." I find the whole approach very degrading and do not recommend it to my patients. Nonetheless, I know of several people who have tried such methods as fasting; ingesting large amounts of every type of fiber from flax seeds to hemp bars, seaweed, and vitamins and minerals; and having the colon flushed out (also known as "colonics") to help them lose weight and "feel better." Most felt distinctly worse for their experience and did not lose any weight. These types of treatment seem to assume that being fat is a character flaw for which people need to be punished. When patients are adequately treated medically and pharmacologically, they do not go looking for these types of treatments.

There was a vogue some years ago for using human chorionic gonadotropin (HCG) injections to help weight loss. Several doctors doing this sort of thing were eventually told by the College of Physicians and Surgeons that it amounted to malpractice because it could cause or enlarge ovarian cysts and was useless for weight loss. In the late 1980s the practice was banned as potentially dangerous. However, the doctors involved changed their approach and went on to run clinics handing out very low-calorie diets that were nutritionally inadequate, accompanying this "therapy" with very high-dose injections of vitamin B-12. So far as we know, this vitamin is harmless; however, it is also quite ineffective in promoting weight loss. People who went to these "diet clinics" lost weight because they were on 500-calorie-a-day diets, not because of the vitamin injections. This approach has been totally discredited. Unfortunately, however, these doctors still do a thriving business.

Use of Laxatives to Lose Weight

This "weight-loss strategy" is based on the myth that laxatives will push food out of the bowel before the calories can be absorbed. Large doses of laxative were seen as a sort of "morning-after" remedy to undo the damage of a binge or a day of excessive overeating. There is no basis in fact for this belief. Not only do laxatives not prevent absorption of calories, they cause loss of essential minerals and water. If you use them often enough, you risk deficiencies of several minerals and vitamins, deficiencies that can have serious side effects such as dehydration and cardiac arrhythmia. Osteoporosis is another risk in the longer term. Laxatives are also addictive, and it is very hard to stop using them once the bowel is dependent on them for normal functioning because without them, constipation and bloating can be very troublesome for months.

Postscript

I hope this book will be helpful to you in a number of ways. It is intended, for one thing, to convince you that problems with weight can be very complex and may require professional help and a multifaceted approach. Above all, however, I hope it will encourage you to insist on the kind of help that is tailored to your own *unique* needs.

Whether you visit a weight-loss clinic, buy a book that contains a weight-loss plan, or see a nutritionist, you can ensure that you receive appropriate help by keeping the following in mind:

1. Be willing to explore and to discover why you are having trouble with weight. Recognize that the reason is almost certainly not that you are eating too much out of sheer self-indulgence or ignorance.

2. Question whether the approach being offered has a methodology that will help you determine what particular factors are interfering with your ability to control food intake.

3. Remember that success in losing weight comes in stages.

   Stage one involves dealing satisfactorily with as many of the contributing medical and emotional problems as possible. This means that you may spend several months getting relief for a sleeping problem, or heartburn due to hiatus hernia, or arthritic pain, depression, anxiety, and so on. Also, because so few people can ignore job issues and relationships in order to make weight loss the number-one priority in their lives, it is impossible to attack weight loss to the exclusion of these other items. During this period you have to become aware of what the weight loss is connected to at a core level. As I mentioned in the introduction, after medical issues are dealt with, the key to weight loss is finding a meaningful reason to lose weight and not being afraid to change.

   Stage two occurs when you have managed your affairs to allow eating to happen at scheduled times, roughly every four hours, rather than randomly. For example, if breakfast is at 8:00 a.m., then lunch or a simple snack has to be eaten at 12:00 noon, even if lunch will be ready at 1:00 p.m. If lunch is at 1:00 p.m., then a snack should be eaten at 5:00 p.m. even though dinner is planned for 6:30 p.m.

   Stage three is reached when you rediscover the ability to differentiate between hunger and other feeling states, such as anger or frustration, and when you also learn to stop eating before you feel full because you can distinguish between the onset of feelings of fullness and complete fullness itself.

   The last stage occurs when you are able to find ways to moderate stress. You also feel in control of other issues that previously caused you to increase your food intake, and you have become physically active.

4. Remember that there are no medications, metabolic stimulants, herbal remedies, or other agents that will accelerate

weight loss successfully where basic medical problems have not been addressed satisfactorily. And above all, remember that medically safe, lasting, weight loss *takes time*.

I wish you success on your journey.

Appendices

Appendix 1: Diagnostic Criteria for Anorexia Nervosa and Bulimia Nervosa

Anorexia Nervosa

1. Refusal to maintain body weight at or above a minimally normal weight for age, sex, and height (subject's weight is generally less than 85 percent of the predicted normal weight).
2. Intense fear of gaining weight or becoming fat, even though underweight.
3. Disturbance in the way in which subject's body weight or shape is experienced, undue influence of body weight or shape on self-evaluation, or denial of the seriousness of the current low body weight.
4. In post-menarchal females, the absence of at least three consecutive menstrual cycles (amenorrhea). A woman is considered to have amenorrhea if her periods occur only following hormone replacement (i.e., oral contraceptive pill).

Bulimia Nervosa

1. Recurrent episodes of binge eating defined as:
   – eating within a two-hour period, an amount of food that is considerably larger than most people would eat during a similar period of time and under similar circumstances;
   – experiencing a lack of control over eating during the episode (e.g., a feeling that one cannot stop eating or control how much one is eating.).
2. Recurrent inappropriate compensatory behavior in order to prevent weight gain, such as self-induced vomiting; misuse of laxatives, diuretics, enemas, or other medications; fasting; or excessive exercise.
3. The binge eating and inappropriate compensatory behaviors both occur, on average, at least twice a week for three months.
4. Self-evaluation is unduly influenced by body shape and weight.
5. The disturbance does not occur exclusively during the episode of bulimia nervosa.

SOURCE: Reprinted with permission from the *Diagnostic and Statistical Manual of Mental Disorders*, Fourth Edition. Copyright 1994 American Psychiatric Association.

Appendix 2: The Harris–Benedict Equations

Basal Energy Expenditure* or Basal Metabolic Rate (BMR), calculations using the Harris–Benedict equations:

Men: $66 + (13.7 \times \text{ideal weight in kg}) + (5 \times \text{height in cm}) - (6.8 \times \text{age in yrs}) = \text{calories required}$

Women: $655 + (9.6 \times \text{ideal weight in kg}) + (1.7 \times \text{height in cm}) - (4.7 \times \text{age in yrs}) = \text{calories required}$

(1 pound = 0.454 kg; 1 inch = 2.54 cm)

*Calorie energy needed to maintain current weight assuming subject is fasting and lying down resting quietly.

Appendix 3: Nomograph for Estimating Body Mass Index (kg/m²)

Directions for Use: Place a ruler or straight edge so that it touches your weight and height as shown in the example. Read off your BMI and see whether it is in an acceptable range or not. Here the ruler intersects a weight of 77 kg and a height of 178 cm giving a BMI of 25.2, which is just acceptable for men.

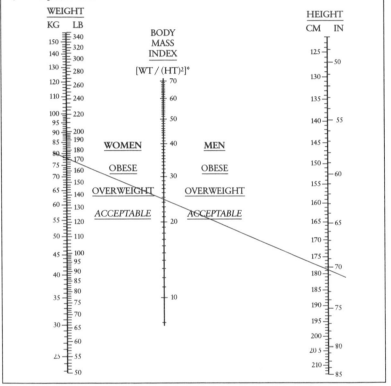

*The ratio of weight/height² emerges from varied epidemiologic studies as the most generally useful index of relative body mass in adults. This nomograph facilitates use of this relationship in clinical situations. While showing the range of weight given as desirable in life insurance studies, the scale expresses relative weight as a continuous variable. This method encourages use of clinical judgment in interpreting "overweight" and "underweight" and in accounting for muscular and skeletal contributions to measured mass.

SOURCE: From G.A. Bray, 1978.

Appendix 4(a): Height-Weight Tables (Metric Units), 1983

This table is useful for determining if your weight is in the correct range, provided you have measured frame size (using one or more methods such as elbow breadth).

HEIGHT (cm)	SMALL FRAME (kg)	MEN MEDIUM FRAME (kg)	LARGE FRAME (kg)	HEIGHT (cm)	SMALL FRAME (kg)	WOMEN MEDIUM FRAME (kg)	LARGE FRAME (kg)
157.5	58.2–60.9	59.4–64.1	62.7–68.2	147.5	46.4–50.5	49.5–55.0	53.6–59.5
160	59.1–61.8	60.5–65.0	63.6–69.5	150	46.8–51.4	50.5–55.9	54.5–60.9
162.5	60.0–62.7	61.4–65.9	64.5–70.9	152.5	47.3–52.3	51.4–57.3	55.5–62.3
165	60.9–63.7	62.3–67.3	65.5–72.7	155	48.2–53.6	52.3–58.6	56.8–63.6
167.5	61.8–64.5	63.2–68.6	66.4–74.5	157.5	49.1–55.0	53.6–60.0	58.2–65.0
170	62.7–65.9	64.5–70.0	67.7–76.4	160	50.5–56.4	55.0–61.4	59.5–66.8
173	63.6–67.3	65.9–71.4	69.1–78.2	162.5	51.8–57.7	56.4–62.7	60.9–68.6
175	64.5–68.6	67.3–72.7	70.5–80.0	165	53.2–59.1	57.7–64.1	62.3–70.5
178	65.4–70.0	68.6–74.1	71.8–81.8	167.5	54.5–60.5	59.1–65.5	63.6–72.3
180	66.4–71.4	70.0–75.5	73.2–83.6	170	55.9–61.8	60.5–66.8	65.0–74.1
183	67.7–72.7	71.4–77.3	74.5–85.6	173	57.3–63.2	61.8–68.2	66.4–75.9
185.5	69.1–74.5	72.7–79.1	76.4–87.3	175	58.6–64.5	63.2–69.5	67.7–77.3
188	70.5–76.4	74.5–80.9	78.2–89.5	178	60.0–65.9	64.5–70.9	69.1–78.6
190.5	71.8–78.2	75.9–82.7	80.0–91.8	180	61.4–67.3	65.9–72.3	70.5–80.0
193	73.6–80.0	77.7–85.0	82.3–94.1	183	62.3–68.6	67.3–73.6	71.8–81.4

The values are statistical computations from individuals ranging from 25 to 59 years of weights by height and body frame at which mortality has been found to be lowest or longevity the highest. Metropolitan Life does not advocate the use of the term "ideal," which has different meanings to various individuals, because the term was used originally in their 1942 to 1943 tables. If one wishes to use these tables in the sense that they are "ideal" in terms of lowest mortality, they are "appropriate" in that context. These tables do not provide weights related to minimizing illness, optimizing job performance, or creating the best appearance.

SOURCE: The 1983 Metropolitan Height-Weight Tables are based on the 1979 Build Study.

Appendix 4(b): Median Heights and Weights and Recommended Energy Intake in the United States

This table gives the average height and weight (i.e., the 50th centile) for men and women at various ages. It shows what their resting energy expenditure (REE) would be and shows a multiplier factor (i.e., 1.50) to get the average energy allowance predicted.

Category	Age (years) or condition	Weight (kg)	Weight (lb)	Height (cm)	Height (in)	Ree[b] (kcal/day)	Multiples of Ree	Energy Allowance (kcal)[c] Per kg	Per day[d]
Infants	0.0–0.5	6	13	60	24	320		108	650
	0.5–1.0	9	20	71	28	500		98	850
Children	1–3	13	29	90	35	740		102	1,300
	4–6	20	44	112	44	950		90	1,800
	7–10	28	62	132	52	1,130		70	2,000
Males	11–14	45	99	157	62	1,440	1.70	55	2,500
	15–18	66	145	176	69	1,760	1.67	45	3,000
	19–24	72	160	177	70	1,780	1.67	40	2,900
	25–50	79	174	176	70	1,800	1.60	37	2,900
	51+	77	170	173	68	1,530	1.50	30	2,300
Females	11–14	46	101	157	62	1,310	1.67	47	2,200
	15–18	55	120	163	64	1,370	1.60	40	2,200
	19–24	58	128	164	65	1,350	1.60	38	2,200
	25–50	63	138	163	64	1,380	1.55	36	2,200
	51+	65	143	160	63	1,280	1.50	30	1,900
Pregnant	1st trimester								+0
	2nd trimester								+300
	3rd trimester								+300
Lactating	1st 6 months								+500
	2nd 6 months								+500

[a]Median Height/Weight used by the RDA are those that are the medians for the U.S. population of designated age as reported in NHANES II.
[b]Calculations based on WHO equation derived from BMR data (Table A–7a), then rounded.
[c]In the range of light to moderate activity, the coefficient of variation is ±20%.
[d]Figure is rounded.

SOURCE: Reprinted with permission from *National Research Council Recommended Dietary Allowances*. Copyright 1989 by the National Academy of Sciences. Courtesy of the National Academy Press, Washington, D.C.

Appendix 5(a): Physical Growth Percentiles: Girls from 2 to 18 Years

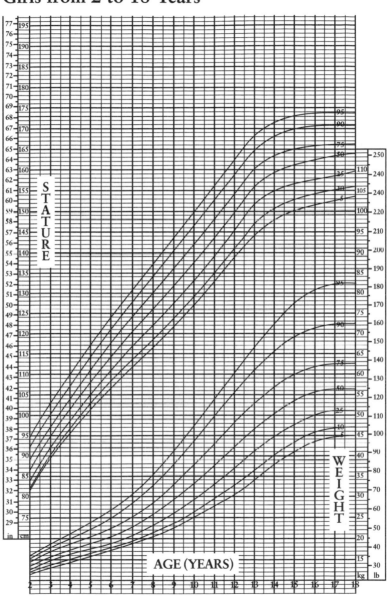

SOURCE: Courtesy of Ross Laboratories, who adapted the growth curves from the orginal data: National Center fro Health Statistics. NCHS Growth Charts, 1976. Monthly Vital Statistics Report, Vol. 25, No. 3. Suppl. (HRA) 76–1120. Rockville, MD, Health Resources Administration, June, 1976. Data from The Fels Research Institute, Yellow Springs, Ohio.

To use this chart:

- **Height percentile:** simply follow a line across from your height to where it meets a line running up from your age. Observe where these two lines intersect on the curved lines graph. Your percentile height is thus determined. For example, if you are 140 cm tall and are 10-1/2 years old, your height is right on the 50th percentile for girls of this age. In other words you are of average height.

- **Weight percentile:** Weight percentile is determined in the same fashion as for height percentile. Simply draw a line vertically upwards from your age until it meets a line running horizontally from your weight. Your weight percentile is thus established. For example, if you are 14 years old and weigh 57 kg, your weight is on the 75th percentile.

Appendix 5(b): Physical Growth Percentiles: Boys from 2 to 18 Years

To use this chart: See instructions for Appendix 3(a).

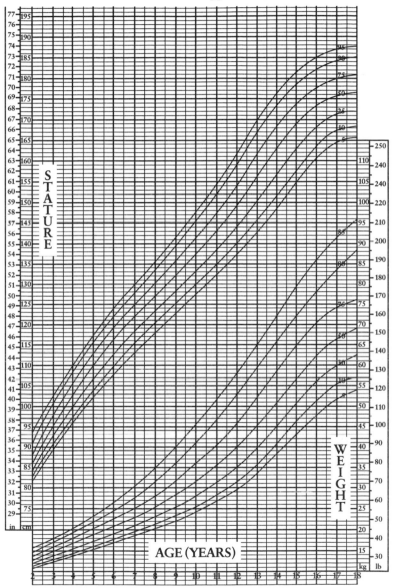

SOURCE: Courtesy of Ross Laboratories, who adapted the growth curves from the orginal data: National Center fro Health Statistics. NCHS Growth Charts, 1976. Monthly Vital Statistics Report, Vol. 25, No. 3. Suppl. (HRA) 76–1120. Rockville, MD, Health Resources Administration, June, 1976. Data from The Fels Research Institute, Yellow Springs, Ohio.

Appendix 6: Frame Size by Elbow Breadth (cm) of United States Male and Female Adults*

This table shows that frame size can be estimated by measuring the distance from the medial epicondyle to the lateral epicondyle of the elbow with calipers.

AGE	FRAME SIZE		
(YEARS)	SMALL	MEDIUM	LARGE
MEN			
18–24	≤6.6	>6.6 AND <7.7	≥7.7
25–34	≤6.7	>6.7 AND <7.9	≥7.9
35–44	≤6.7	>6.7 AND <8.0	≥8.0
45–54	≤6.7	>6.7 AND <8.1	≥8.1
55–64	≤6.7	>6.7 AND <8.1	≥8.1
65–74	≤6.7	>6.7 AND <8.1	≥8.1
WOMEN			
18–24	≤5.6	>5.6 AND <6.5	≥6.5
25–34	≤5.7	>5.7 AND <6.8	≥6.8
35–44	≤5.7	>5.7 AND <7.1	≥7.1
45–54	≤5.7	>5.7 AND <7.2	≥7.2
55–64	≤5.8	>5.8 AND <7.2	≥7.2
65–74	≤5.8	>5.8 AND <7.2	≥7.2

*The tenth and ninetieth percentiles, respectively, represent the predicted mean ±1.282 times the SE. Similarly, the fifteenth and eighty-fifth percentiles are the predicted mean minus and plus, respectively, 1.036 times the SE of the regression equation. There were significant black-white population differences in weight and body composition when age and height were considered. However, when the comparisons were made with reference to age, height, and frame size, there were only minor interpopulation differences. For this reason, all races (white, black, and other) included in the NHANES I and II surveys were merged together for the purpose of calculating percentiles of anthropometric measurements.

S O U R C E : Combined NHANES I and II data sets from A.R. Frisancho, *American Journal of Clinical Nutrition.* Copyright 1984 American society for Clinical Nutrition.

Caliper Application: To measure the distance (cm) between the lateral epicondyle and the medial epicondyle, calipers are applied so that the ends of the caliper fit snugly up against the bony condyles that are just beneath the skin.

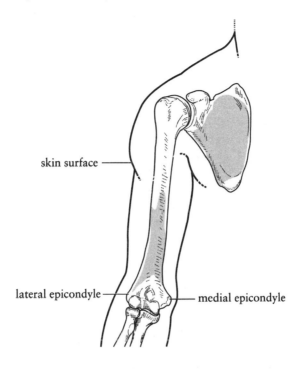

Appendix 7: Recommended Nutrient Intake Based on Age and Body Weight Expressed as Daily Rates

Doctors would refer to this chart to determine whether a person is getting enough of these nutrients. The amounts indicated for each vitamin or mineral are enough to prevent any deficiency syndromes from occurring.

Age	Sex	Weight (kg)	Pro-tein (g)	Vit. A (Re)a (µg)	Vit. D (µg)	Vit. E (mg)	Vit. C (mg)	Fo-late (µg)	Vit. B_{12} (µg)	Cal-cium (mg)	Phos-pho-rus (mg)	Mag-ne-sium (mg)	Iron (mg)	Iodine (µg)	Zinc (mg)
Months															
0–4	Both	6.0	12[b]	400	10	3	20	25	0.3	250[c]	150	20	0.3[d]	30	2[d]
5–12	Both	9.0	12	400	10	3	20	40	0.4	400	200	32	7	40	3
Years															
1	Both	11	13	400	10	3	20	40	0.5	500	300	40	6	55	4
2–3	Both	14	16	400	5	4	20	50	0.6	550	350	50	6	65	4
4–6	Both	18	19	500	5	5	25	70	0.8	600	400	65	8	85	5
7–9	M	25	26	700	2.5	7	25	90	1.0	700	500	100	8	110	7
	F	25	26	700	2.5	6	25	90	1.0	700	500	100	8	95	7
10–12	M	34	34	800	2.5	8	25	120	1.0	900	700	130	8	125	9
	F	36	36	800	2.5	7	25	130	1.0	1100	800	135	8	110	9
13–15	M	50	49	900	2.5	9	30[e]	175	1.0	1100	900	185	10	160	12
	F	48	46	800	2.5	7	30[e]	170	1.0	1000	850	180	13	160	9
16–18	M	62	58	1000	2.5	10	40[e]	220	1.0	900	1000	230	10	160	12
	F	53	47	800	2.5	7	30[e]	190	1.0	700	850	200	12	160	9
19–24	M	71	61	1000	2.5	10	40[e]	220	1.0	800	1000	240	9	160	12
	F	58	50	800	2.5	7	30[e]	180	1.0	700	850	200	13	160	9
25–49	M	74	64	1000	2.5	9	40[e]	230	1.0	800	1000	250	9	160	12
	F	59	51	800	2.5	6	30[e]	185	1.0	700	850	200	13	160	9
50–74	M	73	63	1000	5	7	40[e]	230	1.0	800	1000	250	9	160	12
	F	63	54	800	5	6	30[e]	195	1.0	800	850	210	8	160	9
75+	M	69	59	1000	5	6	40[e]	215	1.0	800	1000	230	9	160	12
	F	64	55	800	5	5	30[e]	200	1.0	800	850	210	8	160	9
Pregnancy (additional)															
1st trimester			5	0	2.5	2	0	200	0.2	500	200	15	0	25	6
2nd trimester			20	0	2.5	2	10	200	0.2	500	200	45	5	25	6
3rd trimester			24	0	2.5	2	10	200	0.2	500	200	45	10	25	6
Lactation (additional)			20	400	2.5	3	25	100	0.2	500	200	65	0	50	6

[a]Retinol Equivalents.
[b]Protein is assumed to be from breast milk and must be adjusted for infant formula.
[c]Infant formula with high phosphorus should contain 375 mg calcium.
[d]Breast milk is assumed to be the source of the mineral.
[e]Smokers should increase vitamin C by 50%.

SOURCE: From Health and Welfare Canada: Nutrition Recommendations. The Report of the Scientific Review Committee. Ottawa, Supply and Services Canada, 1990. Reproduced with permission of the Minister of Supply and Services Canada 1992.

Index